JIMD Reports
Volume 38

Eva Morava
Editor-in-Chief

Matthias Baumgartner · Marc Patterson ·
Shamima Rahman · Johannes Zschocke
Editors

Verena Peters
Managing Editor

JIMD Reports
Volume 38

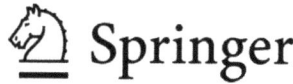 Springer

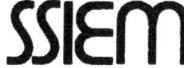

Editor-in-Chief
Eva Morava
Tulane University Medical School
New Orleans
Louisiana
USA

Editor
Matthias Baumgartner
Division of Metabolism & Children's Research
Centre
University Children's Hospital Zürich
Zürich
Switzerland

Editor
Marc Patterson
Division of Child and Adolescent Neurology
Mayo Clinic
Rochester
Minnesota
USA

Editor
Shamima Rahman
Clinical and Molecular Genetics Unit
UCL Institute of Child Health
London
UK

Editor
Johannes Zschocke
Division of Human Genetics
Medical University Innsbruck
Innsbruck
Austria

Managing Editor
Verena Peters
Center for Child and Adolescent Medicine
Heidelberg University Hospital
Heidelberg
Germany

ISSN 2192-8304   ISSN 2192-8312 (electronic)
JIMD Reports
ISBN 978-3-662-56609-1   ISBN 978-3-662-56610-7 (eBook)
https://doi.org/10.1007/978-3-662-56610-7

Contents

First Successful Conception Induced by a Male Cystinosis Patient 1
Koenraad R. Veys, Kathleen W. D'Hauwers, Angelique J. C. M. van Dongen,
Mirian C. Janssen, Martine T. P. Besouw, Ellen Goossens,
Lambert P. van den Heuvel, Alex A. M. M. Wetzels, and Elena N. Levtchenko

Glutaric Acidemia Type 1: A Case of Infantile Stroke 7
Gül Demet Kaya Ozcora, Songul Gokay, Mehmet Canpolat, Fatih Kardaş,
Mustafa Kendirci, and Sefer Kumandaş

Treatment of Depression in Adults with Fabry Disease 13
Nadia Ali, Scott Gillespie, and Dawn Laney

Mutations in *GMPPB* Presenting with Pseudometabolic Myopathy 23
Chiara Panicucci, Chiara Fiorillo, Francesca Moro, Guja Astrea,
Giacomo Brisca, Federica Trucco, Marina Pedemonte, Paola Lanteri,
Lucia Sciarretta, Carlo Minetti, Filippo M. Santorelli, and Claudio Bruno

**Heterogeneous Phenotypes in Lipid Storage Myopathy Due to *ETFDH* Gene
Mutations** 33
Corrado Angelini, Daniela Tavian, and Sara Missaglia

**Successful Management of Pregnancies in Patients with Inherited Disorders
of Ketone Body Metabolism** 41
Raashda Ainuddin Sulaiman, Maha Al-Nemer, Rubina Khan,
Munirah Almasned, Bedour S. Handoum, and Zuhair N. Al-Hassnan

**Improvement of Fabry Disease-Related Gastrointestinal Symptoms
in a Significant Proportion of Female Patients Treated with Agalsidase Beta:
Data from the Fabry Registry** 45
William R. Wilcox, Ulla Feldt-Rasmussen, Ana Maria Martins, Alberto Ortiz,
Roberta M. Lemay, Ana Jovanovic, Dominique P. Germain, Carmen Varas,
Katherine Nicholls, Frank Weidemann, and Robert J. Hopkin

**Ketone Bodies as a Possible Adjuvant to Ketogenic Diet in PDHc Deficiency
but Not in GLUT1 Deficiency** 53
F. Habarou, N. Bahi-Buisson, E. Lebigot, C. Pontoizeau, M. T. Abi-Warde,
A. Brassier, K. H. Le Quan Sang, C. Broissand, S. Vuillaumier-Barrot,
A. Roubertie, A. Boutron, C. Ottolenghi, and P. de Lonlay

GM2 Activator Deficiency Caused by a Homozygous Exon 2 Deletion in *GM2A* . . .   61
Patricia L. Hall, Regina Laine, John J. Alexander, Arunkanth Ankala,
Lisa A. Teot, Hart G. W. Lidov, and Irina Anselm

Effect of Lorenzo's Oil on Hepatic Gene Expression and the Serum Fatty Acid
Level in *abcd1*-Deficient Mice   67
Masashi Morita, Ayako Honda, Akira Kobayashi, Yuichi Watanabe,
Shiro Watanabe, Kosuke Kawaguchi, Shigeo Takashima, Nobuyuki Shimozawa,
and Tsuneo Imanaka

Introduction of a Simple Second Tier Screening Test for C5 Isobars in Dried
Blood Spots: Reducing the False Positive Rate for Isovaleric Acidaemia in
Expanded Newborn Screening   75
R. S. Carling, D. Burden, I. Hutton, R. Randle, K. John, and J. R. Bonham

Open-Label Single-Sequence Crossover Study Evaluating Pharmacokinetics,
Efficacy, and Safety of Once-Daily Dosing of Nitisinone in Patients with
Hereditary Tyrosinemia Type 1   81
Nathalie Guffon, Anders Bröijersén, Ingrid Palmgren, Mattias Rudebeck,
and Birgitta Olsson

A Rapid Two-Step Iduronate-2-Sulfatatse Enzymatic Activity Assay for MPSII
Pharmacokinetic Assessment   89
Mitra Azadeh, Luying Pan, Yongchang Qiu, and Ruben Boado

An Unexplained Congenital Disorder of Glycosylation-II in a Child with
Neurohepatic Involvement, Hypercholesterolemia and Hypoceruloplasminemia . . .   97
Pier Luigi Calvo, Marco Spada, Ivana Rabbone, Michele Pinon,
Francesco Porta, Fabio Cisarò, Stefania Reggiani, Angelo B. Cefalù,
Luisella Sturiale, Domenico Garozzo, Dirk J. Lefeber, and Jaak Jaeken

Peripheral Neuropathy, Episodic Rhabdomyolysis, and Hypoparathyroidism
in a Patient with Mitochondrial Trifunctional Protein Deficiency   101
Peter van Vliet, Annelies E. Berden, Mojca K. M. van Schie, Jaap A. Bakker,
Christian Heringhaus, Irenaeus F. M. de Coo, Mirjam Langeveld,
Marielle A. Schroijen, and M. Sesmu Arbous

JIMD Reports
DOI 10.1007/8904_2017_19

First Successful Conception Induced by a Male Cystinosis Patient

Koenraad R. Veys · Kathleen W. D'Hauwers ·
Angelique J. C. M. van Dongen · Mirian C. Janssen ·
Martine T. P. Besouw · Ellen Goossens ·
Lambert P. van den Heuvel · Alex A. M. M. Wetzels ·
Elena N. Levtchenko

Received: 03 January 2017 / Revised: 06 March 2017 / Accepted: 09 March 2017 / Published online: 13 April 2017
© SSIEM and Springer-Verlag Berlin Heidelberg 2017

Abstract Cystinosis is a rare autosomal recessive lyso-somal storage disease characterized by multi-organ cystine accumulation, leading to renal failure and extra-renal organ dysfunction. Azoospermia of unknown origin is the main cause of infertility in all male cystinosis patients. Although spermatogenesis has shown to be intact at the testicular level in some patients, no male cystinosis patient has been reported yet to have successfully induced conception.

We present the first successful conception ever reported, induced by a 27-year-old male renal transplant infantile nephropathic cystinosis patient through percutaneous epi-didymal sperm aspiration (PESA) followed by intracyto-plasmatic sperm injection (ICSI). After 36 weeks and 6 days of an uncomplicated pregnancy, a dichorial diamniotic (DCDA) twin was born with an appropriate weight for gestational age and in an apparently healthy status. Moreover, we demonstrate that the sperm of epididymal origin in selected male cystinosis patients can be viable for inducing successful conception.

Our observation opens a new perspective in life for many male cystinosis patients whom nowadays have become adults, by showing that despite azoospermia fathering a child can be realized. In addition, our findings raise questions about the possibility of sperm cryopreserva-tion at a young age in these patients.

Communicated by: Robin Lachmann, PhD FRCP

K. R. Veys (✉) · E. N. Levtchenko
Department of Pediatric Nephrology, University Hospitals Leuven, Herestraat 49, 3000 Leuven, Belgium
e-mail: koenraad.veys@uzleuven.be

K. R. Veys · M. T. P. Besouw · L. P. van den Heuvel ·
E. N. Levtchenko
Department of Growth and Regeneration, Unit of Organ Systems, KU Leuven, Herestraat 49, 3000 Leuven, Belgium

K. W. D'Hauwers
Department of Urology, Radboud University Medical Center, Philips van Leydenlaan 15, 6562 EX Nijmegen, The Netherlands

A. J. C. M. van Dongen
Department of Gynaecology, Radboud University Medical Center, Philips van Leydenlaan 15, 6562 EX Nijmegen, The Netherlands

M. C. Janssen
Department of Internal Medicine, Unit of Metabolic Diseases, Radboud University Medical Center, Philips van Leydenlaan 15, 6562 EX Nijmegen, The Netherlands

E. Goossens
Department of Reproduction, Biology of the Testis, Genetics and Regenerative Medicine, Vrije Universiteit Brussel, Laarbeeklaan 103, 1090 Brussels, Belgium

A. A. M. M. Wetzels
Department of Fertility, Radboud University Medical Center, Philips van Leydenlaan 15, 6562 EX Nijmegen, The Netherlands

Introduction

Cystinosis (OMIM #219800) is a rare, autosomal recessive lysosomal storage disease, caused by mutations in the *CTNS* gene encoding cystinosin, a lysosomal proton-cystine cotransporter (Town et al. 1998). It is characterized by lysosomal cystine accumulation and crystal formation in all organs and tissues (Town et al. 1998; Gahl et al. 2002).

The disease initially affects the kidneys, causing renal Fanconi syndrome in early childhood, and progresses to end-stage renal disease in puberty or early adulthood. However, during the first decades of life, various endocrine organs can also be affected (Chan et al. 1970; Fivush et al. 1987, 1988). In addition to primary hypothyroidism,

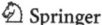

growth retardation, and pancreatic insufficiency, hypergonadotropic hypogonadism has been reported as a frequent finding in male cystinosis patients (Chik et al. 1993). As of yet, in contrast to a few female patients who have given birth, no male cystinosis patient is known to have induced pregnancy. More recently, it was shown that this infertility in male cystinosis patients is due to azoospermia of yet unknown origin (Besouw et al. 2010).

Treatment with the cystine-depleting drug cysteamine delays the onset of end-stage renal disease and prevents multi-organ damage (Markello et al. 1993; Brodin-Sartorius et al. 2012). While first described in 1976 (Thoene et al. 1976), the use of cysteamine in cystinosis patients only became widespread in the early 1990s with the availability of the commercial preparation of cysteamine bitartrate (Cystagon®) (Schneider et al. 1995). Currently, a growing population of cystinosis patients who were treated with cysteamine starting from infancy or early childhood is reaching young adulthood. This prolonged life expectancy raises novel quality of life issues such as male infertility. Here, for the first time ever, we report a successful conception induced by epididymal sperm of a male cystinosis patient through assisted reproductive technology (ART).

Case Report

A 27-year-old male nephropathic cystinosis patient and his wife were consulted at the fertility clinic for realizing their wish of having children.

The patient was formerly diagnosed with nephropathic cystinosis at the age of 4 years when he presented with renal Fanconi syndrome and photophobia. Slit lamp examination revealed the presence of corneal cystine crystals. The diagnosis of cystinosis was confirmed by genetic analysis of the *CTNS* gene showing a compound heterozygous mutation (the common 57 kb deletion on one allele, and a point mutation in the lariat branch site of intron 4: c.141-24T>C on the other allele). The latter mutation results in skipping of exon 5 during transcription (Taranta et al. 2010). The leucocyte cystine level at the moment of diagnosis was 7.8 nmol 1/2 cystine/mg protein. Ever since the initiation of treatment, the total dose of cysteamine has been between 1.3 and 1.9 g/m²/day. End-stage renal disease was developed by the age of 10 years requiring renal replacement therapy (RRT) in the form of peritoneal dialysis. Deceased donor kidney transplantation was followed at the age of 11. The immunosuppressive regimen consisted of ciclosporin A, azathioprine, and low-dose prednisone. Both growth and pubertal development were delayed. At the age of 15, the Tanner stages of puberty were A1P2G2. Height was 153.5 cm, which is below −2 standard deviations (SD), and bone age lagged behind 2 years in comparison to calendar age. Recombinant human growth hormone (rhGH) therapy was initiated after kidney transplantation and resulted in a catch-up growth and a final height of 176 cm. At the age of 18 years, the patient reached a full sexual maturation with Tanner stage 5 and a final bilateral testes volume of 18 mL with a normal consistence. In addition, thyroid function tests always remained within the normal range. Until now, no signs of renal transplant rejection have ever occurred and current eGFR is 110 mL/min/1.73 m².

A previous fertility status evaluation at the age of 21 years showed normal levels of FSH, LH, testosterone, and inhibin B (Table 1, first column). However, no sperm was present in the ejaculate obtained by masturbation, which led to the diagnosis of azoospermia.

Following the consultation at the fertility clinic, the pituitary-testicular axis hormonal status was reassessed

Table 1 Hormonal levels of the pituitary-testicular axis in the reported male cystinosis patient

Age (years)	Ref. value	21	22	22	23	26	27
FSH (U/L)	1.5–11.0	7.79	5.5	6.3	7.4	8.3	8.4
Inhibin B (pg/L)	150–400	210					174
LH (U/L)	1.4–8.5	7.44	4.6	7.4	10.0[a]	7.4	7.3
Testosterone (nmol/L)	11–45	16	9.5	21.6	30.3	15	17
Creatinine (μmol/L)	60–110	83	96	93	100	109	115
Leucocyte cystine level (nmol 1/2 cystine/mg protein)	<1	0.96	2.9	2.42	1.42	2.14	0.78
Cysteamine dose		1,050 mg qid					

Results are reported from the first fertility assessment at the age of 21 years (first column; reported as patient 2 in Besouw et al. (2010)), until the assessment at the age of 27 years prior to the first percutaneous epididymal aspiration (PESA) procedure (last column)

[a] Above the upper normal limit. Based on these results, no primary hypogonadism can be observed. The ejaculate showed azoospermia at the age of 21 and 27 years (data not shown)

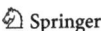

(Table 1, last column). Because of proven azoospermia, and in order to avoid complications related to testicular sperm extraction (TESE), a percutaneous epididymal sperm aspiration (PESA) was performed. The funiculus was anesthetized with prilocaine hydrochloride (Citanest®) and 0.25 mL of epididymal fluid was aspirated on the left side, and 0.5 mL on the right side. This procedure revealed the bilateral presence of mature spermatozoa. In total, from the left epididymis 0.2×10^6 spermatozoa were harvested $(0.80 \times 10^6/mL)$; the right epididymis yielded 2.5×10^6 spermatozoa $(5.0 \times 10^6/mL)$. In both sides, 1% of the spermatozoa showed progressive motility, and 8% showed nonprogressive motility. The sperm was mixed with Test Yolk Buffer (Irvine Scientific, USA) and cryopreserved in abidance of an intracytoplasmatic sperm injection (ICSI) procedure.

In the first ICSI attempt, two oocytes (metaphase II) were obtained, of which one was fertilized. In the second attempt, six out of seven oocytes were fertilized. Single embryo transfer did not result into pregnancy and cryopreservation of the remaining embryos was not possible due to insufficient quality.

A new PESA procedure was performed before the third ICSI attempt. Fifty thousand spermatozoa were obtained from the right epididymis (aspirated total epididymal fluid: 0.5 mL; concentration of spermatozoa: $0.10 \times 10^6/mL$), with 12% progressive and 14% nonprogressive motility. The semen was again cryopreserved. In the third attempt, eight oocytes could be obtained of which six were fertilized. Double embryo transfer was followed on day 3. One embryo was suitable for cryopreservation on day 5 (blastocyst). Two weeks later, a pregnancy test resulted positive, and at 7 weeks of gestation an intact dichorial diamniotic (DCDA) twin was identified by ultrasound. Pregnancy was monitored in a regional hospital and at a gestational age of 36 weeks and 6 days the DCDA twin was born via an uncomplicated caesarean section. Both newborns were apparently healthy with respective birth weights of 2,910 g (son) and 2,884 g (daughter). Subsequently, DNA analysis of the cord blood showed the heterozygous c.141-24T>C mutation in the *CTNS* gene in both offspring, confirming the paternity of our cystinosis patient.

Discussion

Over the last few decades, the advent and progress in cystine-depleting treatment and RRT have significantly improved the prognosis of cystinosis patients (Gahl et al. 2002; Markello et al. 1993; Brodin-Sartorius et al. 2012). As a result of earlier diagnosis, rapid initiation of adequate cysteamine therapy, and improved therapeutic monitoring,

the life expectancy of cystinosis patients has been greatly extended, allowing them nowadays to survive into adulthood.

This favorable evolution has created a new perspective, raising specific adult-related issues. Hence, being one of the essential human needs and major determinants of quality of life, having children has become a matter of concern to adult cystinosis patients and their families.

Here, for the first time, we report a successful conception induced by a male cystinosis patient through ART with PESA followed by ICSI. The paternity of our patient could be confirmed as both offspring inherited the rare heterozygous mutation in the *CTNS* gene, which has only been described in the index case and his sister thus far (Taranta et al. 2010). In addition to the previous report of Besouw et al. which has shown intact spermatogenesis at the testicular level (Besouw et al. 2010), we demonstrate for the first time that the sperm of epididymal origin can be viable in selected male cystinosis patients and can be used for inducing conception successfully.

To this date, the exact pathophysiology of the primary hypogonadism and azoospermia observed in patients with cystinosis is not yet fully understood. In a first organized report on reproductive function in male infantile nephropathic cystinosis patients after renal transplantation published in 1993, hypergonadotropic hypogonadism was shown to be present in the majority of patients (70%) (Chik et al. 1993). This finding could neither be explained by the effect of the previous chronic renal insufficiency nor by renal transplantation and immunosuppressive agents used in the established regimens. In a more recent study, the pituitary-testicular axis remained within normal limits in a subset of male patients although azoospermia was present in all of them (Besouw et al. 2010). Surprisingly, a testicular biopsy in one of these patients showed an intact spermatogenesis (Johnsen score 8–9) (Besouw et al. 2010; Johnsen 1970). As azoospermia was also present in patients treated with cysteamine starting from early age, it remained uncertain whether cysteamine had no therapeutic effect on the pathophysiology of azoospermia, or the drug itself would be involved in causing infertility. In addition, as azoospermia was documented in some patients in the presence of a normal renal function (eGFR), altered renal function cannot be regarded as a major determinant of fertility status (Besouw et al. 2010).

Some hypothetical causes for this azoospermia in nephropathic cystinosis patients with a normal pituitary-testicular axis and renal function can be suggested. First, as spermatogenesis at the testicular level has shown to be intact, it could be hypothesized that epididymal sperm maturation is altered. Epididymal sperm maturation is a process in which spermatozoa acquire their motility and fertilizing capacity during transit from caput to cauda

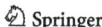

epididymis (Dacheux and Dacheux 2013). This is a crucial step in the establishment of male fertility. Herein, the composition and changing biochemical properties (water, sodium, potassium, bicarbonate, pH, calcium, and osmolality) of the epididymal luminal fluid play a vital role (Dacheux and Dacheux 2013; Pholpramool et al. 2011; Pastor-Soler et al. 2005; Weissgerber et al. 2011). The renal proximal tubule and the epididymis share the same embryonic precursor – the intermediate mesoderm – both are highly metabolically active and serve a shared goal of maintaining electrolyte and acid–base homeostasis through similar transepithelial transport processes. Therefore, although – in contrast to the renal proximal tubule – the sensitivity of epididymal tubular epithelial cells to cystinosin dysfunction is unknown, one could speculate that epididymal transepithelial electrolyte transport in cystinosis is impaired. Indeed, altered acidification of the epididymal luminal fluid milieu has been recognized as a cause of infertility (Pholpramool et al. 2011; Pastor-Soler et al. 2005). In addition, although the exact role of the epididymal luminal Ca^{2+} is not fully clear, the motility and viability of sperm of the cauda epididymis was markedly reduced in a vanilloid type transient receptor potential cation channel 6 knock-out ($trpv6^{-/-}$) murine model, in the presence of abnormal high calcium concentrations in the intraluminal fluid of the cauda epididymis (Weissgerber et al. 2011).

Second, in vivo and in vitro data on cysteamine, being the only available disease-modifying drug, suggest an indirect local as well as a systemic endocrine effect, the latter through actions of ghrelin. Via inhibition of somatostatin secretion, cysteamine increases plasma ghrelin levels (Fukuhara et al. 2005). Ghrelin has shown to exert a central inhibitory effect on FSH and LH secretion, as well as a local inhibitory effect on Leydig cell proliferation and testosterone secretion (Comninos et al. 2014). In addition, cysteamine can potentially induce alterations of posttranslational modifications in epididymal sperm (Sutovsky 2014). Furthermore, a spermicide effect of cysteamine has been documented by a moderate reversible inhibition of human acrosin, a protease which is released from the acrosome of the spermatozoa in the acrosome reaction, which is crucial to the penetration of the zona pellucida (Anderson et al. 1998). However, whether cysteamine penetrates the blood–testes barrier and which concentrations can be reached in the human sperm is currently unknown.

Cystine crystal deposits and signs of increased fibrosis have been previously demonstrated in testes in an infantile nephropathic cystinosis patient under cysteamine therapy (Chik et al. 1993). However, in this case, the patient had clear signs of primary hypogonadism, sufficient to explain his infertility. As several studies demonstrated recently that cystinosin is involved in numerous cellular processes, one

can argue whether merely the lysosomal cystine accumulation should be considered as the only pathophysiological mechanism involved in infertility (Raggi et al. 2014; Giade Chevronnay et al. 2015; Ivanova et al. 2015, 2016; Rega et al. 2016). In this regard, it is of note that the cystinosin-LKG isoform, of which its localization is not limited to the lysosomal membrane, has the highest expression in the testes compared to other organs (Taranta et al. 2008). Obviously, further research is needed in order to unravel the underlying mechanism of the azoospermia observed in male cystinosis patients. In the meanwhile, ART can help these patients to realize their wish of having children.

As an important subset of male cystinosis patients have been described to evolve into a primary hypogonadism as early as the second decade of life, sperm cryopreservation in pubertal male cystinosis patients could be considered to maximize their chances on fathering a child. PESA offers the advantage of avoiding complications related to sperm retrieval techniques at the testicular level. Moreover, the success rate of a surgical sperm retrieval technique, like PESA, followed by ICSI, is non-inferior in comparison to the regular in vitro fertilization (IVF) with ejaculated semen (Gozlan et al. 2007). It remains uncertain however, whether the ejaculate of pubertal boys with cystinosis will contain sperm cells that can be used for cryopreservation at all, since this has never been tested before. Obviously, the optimal timing at which cryopreservation would have to be performed will raise ethical dilemmas and may also verge on the borders of current scientific and practical feasibility. Because of the vulnerability of this age group, the potential emotional impact of fertility preservation and the ethical concerns, psychological counseling should be a regular part of a multidisciplinary team, experienced in guiding patients through the cryopreservation and ART procedures. Ultimately, the most important ethical justification for considering fertility preservation techniques in cystinosis patients is to serve their best interests and universal needs in life.

Taken together, this first successful conception induced by a male cystinosis patient may be considered as a milestone and the dawn of a new era for the entire cystinosis community.

Acknowledgements We would like to express our gratitude to the treating gynecologist at the regional hospital, Fleurisca Korteweg, for the meticulous follow-up of the pregnancy, to professor emeritus Leo Monnens for carefully revising the manuscript and his particularly appreciated advice, and to the Cystinosis Research Foundation Ireland for funding this research.

Take-Home Message

The first successful conception induced by a male cystinosis patient, whom are known to have azoospermia of

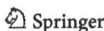

unknown origin, introduces the dawn of a new era for all patients with this previously fatal metabolic disease.

Details of the Contributions of Individual Authors

The Abstract, Introduction, and Discussion sections were drafted by K. Veys and carefully revised by M. Besouw, E. Goossens, B. van den Heuvel, and E. Levtchenko. The Case Report section was drafted by K. D'Hauwers, A. Van Dongen, M. Janssen, and A. Wetzels, and revised by E. Goossens. Sequencing of the CTNS mutation of the reported patient was performed by B. van den Heuvel. The urologic procedures (PESA) in the reported patient were performed by K. D'Hauwers. The fertilization procedures were coordinated by A. Wetzels. The follow-up of the pregnancy and delivery were managed by A. Van Dongen. M. Janssen and E. Levtchenko are the treating physicians of the cystinosis patient.

Competing Interest Statement

None to declare.

Details of Funding

E. Levtchenko is supported by the Research Foundation – Flanders (F.W.O. Vlaanderen), grant 1801110N, the Cystinosis Research Network and Cystinosis Ireland.

K. Veys is funded by the Research Foundation – Flanders (F.W.O. Vlaanderen), grant 11Y5216N.

Details of Ethical Approval

The procedure was performed as part of regular patient care.

References

Anderson RA Jr, Feathergill K, Kirkpatrick R, Zaneveld LJ, Coleman KT, Spear PG et al (1998) Characterization of cysteamine as a potential contraceptive anti-HIV agent. J Androl 19:37–49

Besouw M, Kremer JA, Janssen MC, Levtchenko EN (2010) Fertility status in male cystinosis patients treated with cysteamine. Fertil Steril 93:1880–1883

Brodin-Sartorius A, Tête MJ, Niaudet P, Antignac C, Guest G, Ottolenghi C et al (2012) Cysteamine therapy delays the progression of nephropathic cystinosis in late adolescents and adults. Kidney Int 81:179–189

Chan AM, Lynch MJ, Bailey JD, Ezrin C, Fraser D (1970) Hypothyroidism in cystinosis. A clinical, endocrinologic and histologic study involving sixteen patients with cystinosis. Am J Med 48:678–692

Chik L, Friedman A, Merriam GR, Gahl WA (1993) Pituitary-testicular function in nephropathic cystinosis. Ann Intern Med 119:568–575

Comninos AN, Jayasena CN, Dhillo WS (2014) The relationship between gut and adipose hormones and reproduction. Hum Reprod Update 20:153–174

Dacheux JL, Dacheux F (2013) New insights into epididymal function in relation to sperm maturation. Reproduction 147:2742

Fivush B, Green OC, Porter CC, Balfe JW, O'Regan S, Gahl WA (1987) Pancreatic endocrine insufficiency in posttransplant cystinosis. Am J Dis Child 141:1087–1089

Fivush B, Flick JA, Gahl WA (1988) Pancreatic exocrine insufficiency in a patient with nephropathic cystinosis. J Pediatr 112:49–51

Fukuhara S, Suzuki H, Masaoka T, Arakawa M, Hosoda H, Minegishi Y et al (2005) Enhanced ghrelin secretion in rats with cysteamine-induced duodenal ulcers. Am J Physiol Gastrointest Liver Physiol 289:138–145

Gahl WA, Thoene JG, Schneider JA (2002) Cystinosis. N Engl J Med 347:111–121

Giade Chevronnay HP, Janssens V, Van Der Smissen P, Liao XH, Abid Y, Nevo N et al (2015) A mouse model suggests two mechanisms for thyroid alterations in infantile cystinosis: decreased thyroglobulin synthesis due to endoplasmic reticulum stress/unfolded protein response and impaired lysosomal processing. Endocrinology 156:2349–2364

Gozlan I, Dor A, Farber B, Meirow D, Feinstein S, Levron J (2007) Comparing intracytoplasmatic sperm injection and in vitro fertilization in patients with single oocyte retrieval. Fertil Steril 87:515–518

Ivanova EA, De Leo MG, Van Den Heuvel L, Pastore A, Dijkman H, De Matteis MA et al (2015) Endo-lysosomal dysfunction in human proximal tubular epithelial cells deficient for lysosomal cystine transporter cystinosin. PLoS One 10:e0120998

Ivanova EA, van den Heuvel LP, Elmonem MA, De Smedt H, Missiaen L, Pastore A et al (2016) Altered mTOR signaling in nephropathic cystinosis. J Inherit Metab Dis 39:457–464

Johnsen SG (1970) Testicular biopsy score count – a method for registration of spermatogenesis in human testes: normal values and results in 335 hypogonadal males. Hormones 1:2–25

Markello TC, Bernardini IM, Gahl WA (1993) Improved renal function in children with cystinosis treated with cysteamine. N Engl J Med 328:1157–1162

Pastor-Soler N, Piétrement C, Breton S (2005) Role of acid/base transporters in the male reproductive tract and potential consequences of their malfunction. Physiology (Bethesda) 20:417–428

Pholpramool C, Borwornpinyo S, Dinudom A (2011) Role of Na$^+$/H$^+$ exchanger 3 in the acidification of the male reproductive tract and male fertility. Clin Exp Pharmacol Physiol 38:403–409

Raggi C, Luciani A, Nevo N, Antignac C, Terryn S, Devuyst O (2014) Dedifferentiation and aberrations of the endolysosomal compartment characterize the early stage of nephropathic cystinosis. Hum Mol Genet 23:2266–2278

Rega LR, Polishchuk E, Montefusco S, Napolitano G, Tozzi G, Zhang J et al (2016) Activation of the transcription factor EB rescues lysosomal abnormalities in cystinotic kidney cells. Kidney Int 89:862–873

Schneider JA, Clark KF, Greene AA, Reisch JS, Markello TC, Gahl WA et al (1995) Recent advances in the treatment of cystinosis. J Inherit Metab Dis 18:387–397

Sutovsky P (2014) Posttranslational protein modifications in the reproductive system. In: Sutovsky P (ed) Advances in experimental medicine and biology. Springer, New York, p 759

Taranta A, Petrini S, Palma A, Mannucci L, Wilmer MJ, De Luca V et al (2008) Identification and subcellular localization of a new cystinosin isoform. Am J Physiol Renal Physiol 294:F1101–F1108

Taranta A, Wilmjer MJ, van den Heuvel LP, Bencivenga P, Bellomo F, Levtchenko EN et al (2010) Analysis of CTNS gene transcripts in nephropathic cystinosis. Pediatr Nephrol 25:1263–1267

Thoene JG, Oshima RG, Crawhall JC, Olson DL, Schneider JA (1976) Cystinosis. Intracellular cystine depletion by aminothiols in vitro and in vivo. J Clin Invest 58:180–189

Town M, Jean G, Cherqui S, Attard M, Forestier L, Whitmore SA et al (1998) A novel gene encoding an integral membrane protein is mutated in nephropathic cystinosis. Nat Genet 18:319–324

Weissgerber P, Kriebs U, Tsvilovskyy V, Olausson J, Kretz O, Stoerger C et al (2011) Male fertility depends on Ca^{2+} absorption by TRPV6 in epididymal epithelia. Sci Signal 4:1–13

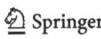

JIMD Reports
DOI 10.1007/8904_2017_26

RESEARCH REPORT

Glutaric Acidemia Type 1: A Case of Infantile Stroke

Gül Demet Kaya Ozcora · Songul Gokay ·
Mehmet Canpolat · Fatih Kardaş · Mustafa Kendirci ·
Sefer Kumandaş

Received: 20 November 2016 / Revised: 30 March 2017 / Accepted: 03 April 2017 / Published online: 15 April 2017
© SSIEM and Springer-Verlag Berlin Heidelberg 2017

Abstract *Background*: Glutaric acidemia Type 1 (GA-1) is an autosomal recessively inherited metabolic disorder which is associated with *GCDH* gene mutations which alters the glutaryl-CoA dehydrogenase, an enzyme playing role in the catabolic pathways of the amino acids lysine, hydroxylysine, and tryptophan. Clinical findings are often encephalopathic crises, dystonia, and extrapyramidal symptoms.

Case Report: A 9-month-old male infant referred to our department with focal tonic-clonic seizures during rotavirus infection and acute infarcts in MRI. Clinical manifestation, MRI findings, and metabolic investigations directed thoughts towards GA-I. Molecular genetic testing revealed a homozygous c.572T>C (p.M191T) mutation in *GCDH* gene which confirmed the diagnosis. Application of protein restricted diet, carnitine and riboflavin supplementations prevented the progression of Magnetic Resonance Imaging (MRI) and clinical pathologic findings during the 1 year of follow-up period.

Conclusion: This case is of great importance since it shows possibility of infantile stroke in GA-1, significance of early diagnosis and phenotypic variability of disease.

Communicated by: Piero Rinaldo, MD, PhD

G. D. Kaya Ozcora (✉) · M. Canpolat · S. Kumandaş
Faculty of Medicine, Department of Pediatrics, Division of Pediatric Neurology, Erciyes University, Kayseri, Turkey
e-mail: guldemetkaya@hotmail.com

S. Gokay · F. Kardaş · M. Kendirci
Division of Pediatric Nutrition and Metabolism, Erciyes University, Kayseri, Turkey

Introduction

Glutaric acidemia Type 1 (GA-1) (OMIM number #231670) is an autosomal recessively inherited, treatable disease which was to be addressed first by Goodman et al. (1975). Mutations in the glutaryl-CoA dehydrogenase (*GCDH*) gene result in glutaryl-CoA dehydrogenase (Enzyme Commission number 1.3.8.6) deficiency which is a key enzyme in the catabolic pathways of the amino acids lysine, hydroxylysine, and tryptophan. The estimated prevalence is 1 in 30,000–100,000 newborns whereas this prevalence might be much higher in some countries with high rates of consanguineous marriages (Tang et al. 2000; Strauss et al. 2003; Kölker et al. 2006, 2011; Baradaran et al. 2014). *GCDH* deficiency is characterized by increased levels of organic acid excretions; namely of glutaric acid, 3-hydroxyglutaric acid (3-OHGA), glutaconic acid in urine and glutarylcarnitine in plasma. Increased urinary concentrations of 3-OHGA is the most sensitive biochemical marker for diagnosis (Al-Dirbashi et al. 2011).

Clinical presentation with acute encephalopathic crises mostly between 6th and 18th months is triggered by febrile illness, fasting, or immunization. As for the discourse of onset, late, slowly progressive and insidious onset of cases have been defined (Fraidakis et al. 2014). Affected patients often present with dystonia and extrapyramidal symptoms such as athetosis, seizures, and intellectual disability. The macrocephaly prevalence in GA-1 is about 75% of the patients (Babu et al. 2015).

In this study, we hereby report a case with GA-1 presented with recurrent brain infarcts. Although metabolic strokes may be seen in patients with isovaleric, methyl malonic, and propionic acidemias, stroke is rarely observed in the presentation of GA-1 (Hoffmann et al. 1994).

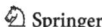

Case

A 9-month-old male infant born out of consanguineous marriage between first cousins admitted with the complaint of focal tonic-clonic seizures during a rotavirus infection. There was no history of asphyxia or trauma. The neurologic and neuropsychological examinations were unremarkable. Biochemical investigations including serum electrolytes, blood glucose, and liver functions were within normal limits. The electroencephalography (EEG) showed normal results, so seizures were evaluated as symptomatic. Due to the focal tonic-clonic seizure episode secondary to infection, MRI of the brain was requested which revealed restricted diffusion consistent with acute infarcts in the bilateral basal ganglia, mildly dilated appearances in the lateral ventricles and an arachnoid cyst in the left Sylvian fissure (Fig. 1). Metabolic diseases screenings and coagulation anomalies were investigated and enoxaparin treatment was initiated and terminated on the 5th day due to the normal coagulation profile. On the 15th day of the hospitalization, a new MRI was ordered due to the weakness in the right-hand which showed a new infarction extending to the internal capsule genus at the level of the left globus pallidus (Fig. 2). Despite the absence of macrocephaly, characteristic presentation and neuroimaging findings along with metabolic investigations suggested the diagnosis of GA-I (Table 1). Molecular genetic testing confirmed that the patient had a homozygous and parents had heterozygous c.572T>C (p. M191T) mutation related to GA-1 which was reported in one

patient from Germany (our case is Turkish) and labeled as likely pathogenic in databases (Schwartz et al. 1998).

The treatment with protein restricted diet (1.4 g/kg/day natural protein, 1 g/kg/day protein with amino acid supplements), carnitine (100 mg/kg/day), and riboflavin (100 mg/day) supplementations was initiated. During the follow-up while patient was on diet, there were no observed metabolic crises even if he had infections, but delayed motor and language development were significant in comparison with his peers. He started to walk without support when he was 24-month-old and currently (38-month-old) speaks only few words and there is still mild right hemiparesis. Because of normal control EEG tests and a seizure-free period antiepileptic treatment was withdrawn after 2 years. Control brain MRI after 29 months from first evaluation showed loss of volume and a T2 signal increase in the left putamen and caudate nucleus, and minimal volume loss and a slight T2 signal increase in the right putamen, and an arachnoid cyst in the left anterior temporal lobe and left anterior frontal lobe (Fig. 3).

Discussion

GA-1 is a treatable neurometabolic disease of autosomal recessive trait which develops due to the mutations of *GCDH* gene on chromosome 19p13. It might prevail more frequently in some populations with high rates of consanguinity and first cousin marriages as in our case. The usual

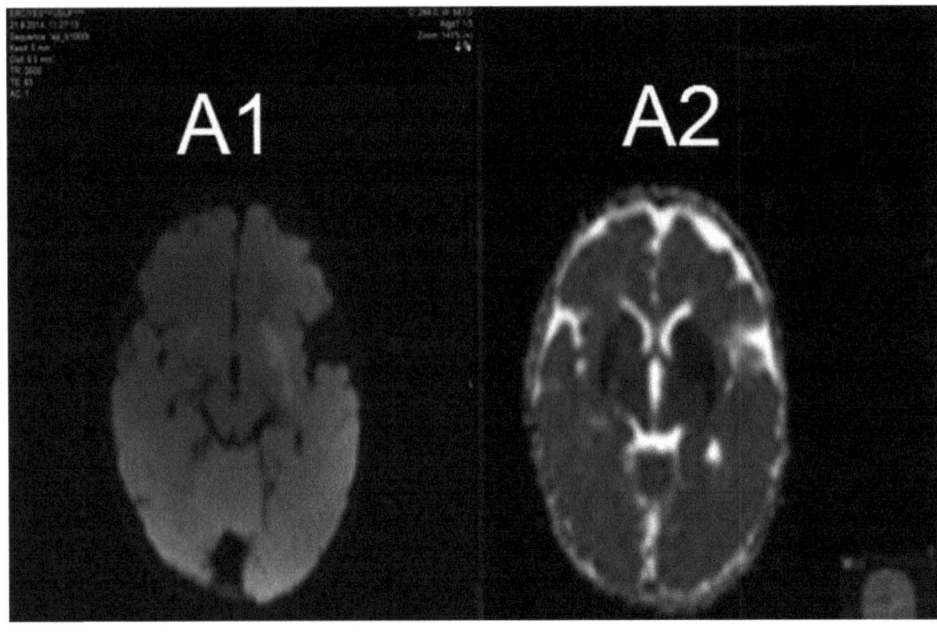

Fig. 1 A1 (diffusion weighted sequences) and A2 (apparent diffusion coefficient); MRI of the brain: restricted diffusion consistent with acute infarcts in the bilateral basal ganglions, mildly dilated appearances in the lateral ventricles and an arachnoid cyst in the left Sylvian fissure

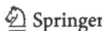

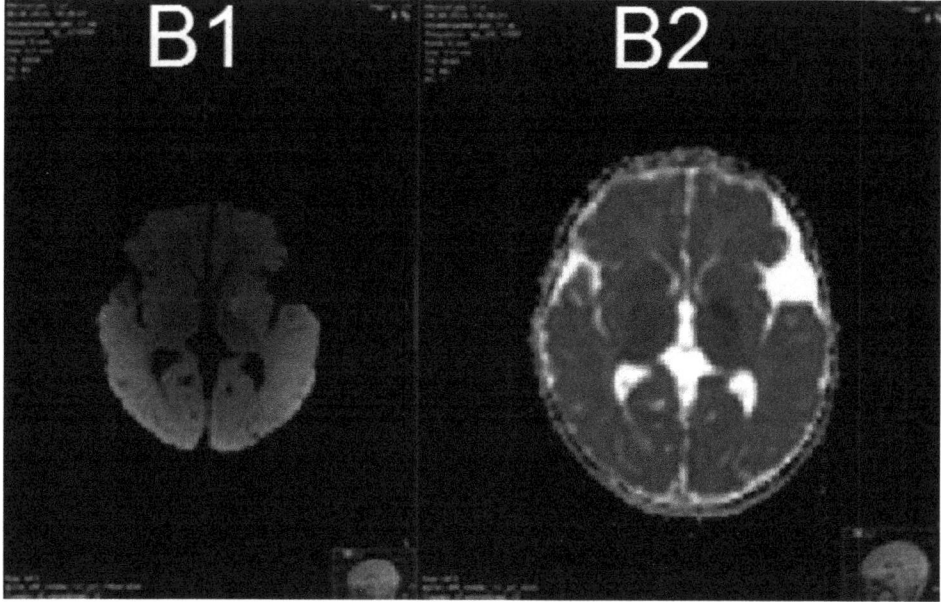

Fig. 2 B1 (diffusion weighted sequences) and B2 (apparent diffusion coefficient); 15 days after from the first brain MRI; A new infarction in the internal capsule genus at the level of the left globus pallidus

Table 1 Blood and urine biochemistry results of case

Metabolite	Result (μmol/L)	Normal (μmol/L)
	Tandem MS	
Free carnitine (C0)	3.07	7.00–80.00
Total carnitine	37	25.0–75.0
Glutaryl carnitine	0.6	0.35–20.0
C5DC/C8	2.87	0.0–1.8
C5DC/C16	0.48	0.0–0.06
	GC-MS	
Glutaric acid (GA)	0	00.0–3.8
3-Hydroxyglutaric	0	00.0–4.6

age of presentation varies from 6 months to 2 years of age; often triggered by an infection, fasting, or immunization with acute metabolic encephalopathy. There may also be acute neuroregression and extrapyramidal symptoms following an initial phase of normal or almost normal development by striatal necrosis with stroke like characteristics. As the disease exhibits a slow progression, late onset presentations or asymptomatic cases in elderly ages were rarely reported (Fraidakis et al. 2014; Wang et al. 2014). Our case is compatible with typical age of presentation with 9 months of age, he was the first child of the family with consanguineous marriage and presented with stroke associated seizure during an acute gastroenteritis.

Due to the bilateral symmetric striatum involvement, impairment of perfusion in both infarcted watershed areas and the absence of the distribution of blood flow derived from the affected blood vessels and clinically silent clinical manifestation in comparison with ischemic stroke patient was with diagnosed metabolic infarction due to glutaric aciduria (Strauss et al. 2007).

Macrocephaly, acute encephalitis like crises, dystonia due to bilateral striatal injury, and characteristic frontotemporal atrophy are the hallmarks of the disease. Generalized dystonia superimposed on axial hypotonia is predominantly occurred following an acute encephalitis crisis. Dystonia and hypotonia were not existed in our case at the time of diagnosis. Macrocephaly is a constant feature and can be present at birth or a rapid increase of head circumference can take place after birth with an estimated frequency of 65–75% reported in patients with GA-1, however microcephaly can be observed in patients with GA-1 during the first 8 months of life and besides there were cases reported

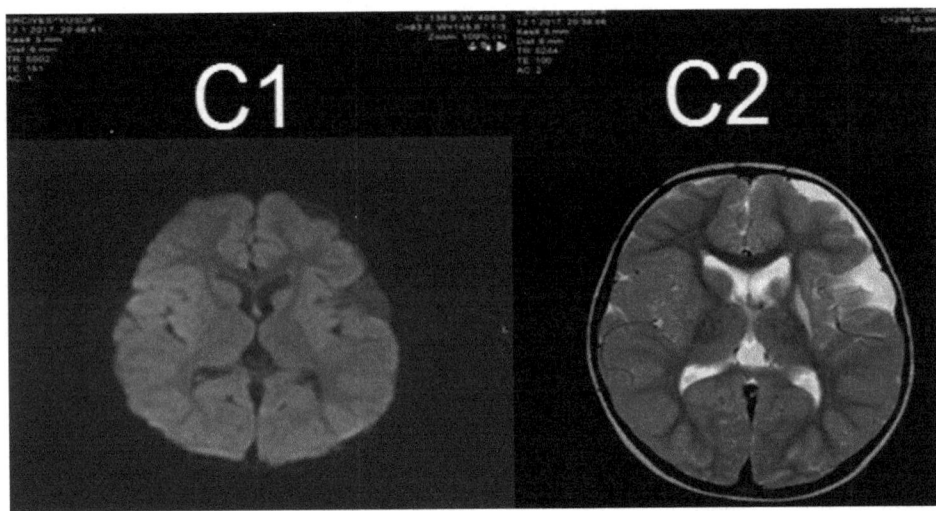

Fig. 3 C1 (diffusion weighted sequences) and C2 (apparent diffusion coefficient); 29 months after from the first MRI; loss of volume and a T2 signal increase in the left putamen and caudate nucleus, and minimal volume loss and a slight T2 signal increase in the right putamen, and an arachnoid cyst in the left anterior temporal lobe and left anterior frontal lobe

without macrocephaly (Baradaran et al. 2014; Gupta et al. 2014; Wang et al. 2014). There is no association between macrocephaly and outcome whereas in some cases the frequency of macrocephaly was higher in mild impairment group than severe one, leading to an early diagnosis by macrocephaly (Mushimoto et al. 2011). In our case the above stated symptoms were all absent except encephalitis like crises, he was normocephalic with occipitofrontal circumference of 50–75th percentile for chronologic age.

Cranial radiologic imaging is generally useful and specific but still lacks high rates of success about diagnosis. Frontotemporal atrophy is the earliest feature, even in the asymptomatic period. Structural changes of basal ganglia, incomplete opercularization of the insular cortex, widening of the Sylvian fissures, and cerebrospinal fluid spaces are the characteristic of GA-1. Deep white matter and diffuse periventricular involvement can be existed for early or late onset subtypes and they seem to be correlated with duration of the disease and are not clinically subtype specific (Bähr et al. 2002). Published data reveals that MRI abnormalities have been defined for all patients with or without clinical signs; the severity of striatal lesions on MRI correlates with severity of the movement disorder and extra-striatal MRI findings do not correlate with the movement disorder (Harting et al. 2009; Garbade et al. 2014; Pusti et al. 2014; Wang et al. 2014). In our case, there was existed striatal injury but no movement disorders such as dystonia.

Up to now, more than 200 mutations have been detected in the *GCDH* gene. R402W and E181Q mutations are more prevalent than the other types (Baradaran et al. 2014; Gupta et al. 2014). There is no data about the types of common genetic mutations responsible for GA-1 in Turkey. Homozygous mutation of c.572T>C (p.M191T) as in our case first was reported in 1998 in a male patient with German origin with <0.5% residual enzyme activity (Schwartz et al. 1998). The disease exhibits clinical variability which has a correlation with differently altered enzymatic activities due to the different positions of pathogenic variants in *GCDH* gene (Gupta et al. 2014). We weren't able to analyze the residual enzyme activity for our case due to financial problems.

Because of parents are heterozygous carriers, during genetic counseling preimplantation genetic diagnosis was explained to family in case of planned pregnancy due to the 25% chance of child to be affected.

In compliance with the findings of previous studies, there is no correlation between phenotype and genotype, but some of the mutations are correlated with the excretion of glutaric acid and residual enzyme activity (Goodman et al. 1975; Baradaran et al. 2014; Gupta et al. 2014). As for our case, there was no urinary excretion of glutaric (GA) and hydroxyglutaric acids (3-OHGA). As the sustained Tandem Mass Spectrometry, high level of C5DC in the repeated tests suggested the existence of GA-1, genetic molecular analysis was recommended out of suspicion for GA-1, even though the outcomes of analysis for organic acids in urine were all normal.

The newborn screening will be beneficial for a better outcome as the diagnostic delay may also lead to irreversible damage. Although it is the case that 10–20% of the patients still develop some level of motor and intellectual impairment (Boy et al. 2016) even with an appropriate treatment, excellent outcomes can be obtained thanks to early diagnosis and dietary therapy nevertheless. Our patient was asymptomatic at 9 months of age; such symptoms as macrocephaly, movement disorder, feeding

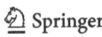

problems, or psychomotor delay were absent. In contrast to the fact reported by the previous data that patients with early onset suffer worse neurological outcome when compared to patients with late onset, our case with early onset happened to involve mildly good neurological outcome (Wang et al. 2014). The neurological development of the patient was close to the normal and there were no recurrent seizures. This clinical case has been reported herein to highlight the phenotypic variability of neuro-metabolic disorders such as GA-I, and emphasize the importance of a high index of suspicion.

Details of the Contributions of Individual Authors

Gül Demet Kaya Ozcora, Mustafa Kendirci, Sefer Kumandaş: collected the data, conducted the analyses and interpretation of the data, and prepared early drafts of the paper.

Gül Demet Kaya Ozcora, Mustafa Kendirci, Sefer Kumandaş: conceptualized and supervised development of the research, assisted with analysis and interpretation of the data and contributed to writing the manuscript.

Gül Demet Kaya Ozcora, Songül Gökay: participated in the collection of the data and helped manuscript preparation.

Mehmet Canpolat, Fatih Kardaş: helped in recruitment and provide testing facilities.

All authors read and approved the final manuscript.

The Name of the Corresponding Author

Gul Demet Kaya Ozcora, MD

Erciyes University Medical School, Department of Pediatrics, Division of Pediatric Neurology, Melikgazi, Kayseri, Turkey

Telephone: +90 352 2076666/0 506 897 5699

Facsimile: +90 352 4375825

E-mail: guldemetkaya@hotmail.com

A Competing Interest Statement

The authors declare that there is no conflict of interest regarding this work.

Conflict of Interest

Gül Demet Kaya Ozcora, Songul Gokay, Mehmet Canpo-lat, Fatih Kardaş, Mustafa Kendirci, Sefer Kumandaş declare that they have no conflict of interest.

Details of Funding

This work received no specific grant from any funding organization.

Ethics Statements

All procedures followed were in accordance with the ethical standards of the responsible committee on human experimentation (institutional and national) and with the Helsinki Declaration of 1975, as revised in 2000. Parents provided informed consent prior to use their child's history information, genetic test results, photographs, and video images. Signed consent form for publication was obtained.

References

Al-Dirbashi OY, Kölker S, Ng D et al (2011) Diagnosis of glutaric aciduria type 1 by measuring 3-hydroxyglutaric acid in dried urine spots by liquid chromatography tandem mass spectrometry. J Inherit Metab Dis 34:173–180

Babu RP, Bishnupriya G, Thushara PK et al (2015) Detection of glutaric acidemia type 1 in infants through tandem mass spectrometry. Mol Genet Metabol Rep 3:75–79

Bähr O, Mader I, Zschocke J, Dichgans J, Schulz J (2002) Adult onset glutaric aciduria type I presenting with a leukoencephalopathy. Neurology 59:1802–1804

Baradaran M, Galehdari H, Aminzadeh M, Azizi Malmiri R, Tangestani R, Karimi Z (2014) Molecular determination of glutaric aciduria type I in individuals from southwest Iran. Arch Iran Med 17:629–632

Boy N, Mühlhausen C, Maier EM et al (2016) Proposed recommendations for diagnosing and managing individuals with glutaric aciduria type I: second revision. J Inherit Metab Dis 40:75–101

Fraidakis M, Liadinioti C, Stefanis L et al (2014) Rare late-onset presentation of glutaric aciduria type I in a 16-year-old woman with a novel GCDH mutation. In: JIMD reports, vol 18. Springer, Berlin, pp 85–92

Garbade SF, Greenberg CR, Demirkol M et al (2014) Unravelling the complex MRI pattern in glutaric aciduria type I using statistical models – a cohort study in 180 patients. J Inherit Metab Dis 37:763–773

Goodman SI, Markey SP, Moe PG, Miles BS, Teng CC (1975) Glutaric aciduria; a "new" disorder of amino acid metabolism. Biochem Med 12:12–21

Gupta N, Singh PK, Kumar M et al (2014) Glutaric acidemia type 1-clinico-molecular profile and novel mutations in GCDH gene in Indian patients. In: JIMD reports, vol 21. Springer, Berlin, pp 45–55

Harting I, Neumaier-Probst E, Seitz A et al (2009) Dynamic changes of striatal and extrastriatal abnormalities in glutaric aciduria type I. Brain 132:1764–1782

Hoffmann G, Gibson K, Tretz F, Nyhan W, Bremer H (1994) Neurological manifestations of organic acid disorders. Eur J Pediatr 153:S94–S100

Kölker S, Garbade SF, Greenberg CR et al (2006) Natural history, outcome, and treatment efficacy in children and adults with glutaryl-CoA dehydrogenase deficiency. Pediatr Res 59:840–847

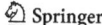

Kölker S, Christensen E, Leonard JV et al (2011) Diagnosis and management of glutaric aciduria type I–revised recommendations. J Inherit Metab Dis 34:677–694

Mushimoto Y, Fukuda S, Hasegawa Y et al (2011) Clinical and molecular investigation of 19 Japanese cases of glutaric acidemia type 1. Mol Genet Metab 102:343–348

Pusti S, Das N, Nayek K, Biswas S (2014) A treatable neurometabolic disorder: glutaric aciduria type 1. Case Rep Pediatr 2014:1–3

Schwartz M, Christensen E, Superti-Furga A, Brandt NJ (1998) The human glutaryl-CoA dehydrogenase gene: report of intronic sequences and of 13 novel mutations causing glutaric aciduria type I. Hum Genet 102:452–458

Strauss KA, Puffenberger EG, Robinson DL, Morton DH (2003) Type I glutaric aciduria, part 1: natural history of 77 patients. Am J Med Genet C Semin Med Genet 121C:38–52

Strauss KA, Lazovic J, Wintermark M, Morton DH (2007) Multimodal imaging of striatal degeneration in Amish patients with glutaryl-CoA dehydrogenase deficiency. Brain 130:1905–1920

Tang NL, Hui J, Law L et al (2000) Recurrent and novel mutations of GCDH gene in Chinese glutaric acidemia type I families. Hum Mutat 16:446–446

Wang Q, Li X, Ding Y, Liu Y, Song J, Yang Y (2014) Clinical and mutational spectra of 23 Chinese patients with glutaric aciduria type 1. Brain Dev 36:813–822

JIMD Reports
DOI 10.1007/8904_2017_21

RESEARCH REPORT

Treatment of Depression in Adults with Fabry Disease

Nadia Ali · Scott Gillespie · Dawn Laney

Received: 02 November 2016 / Revised: 08 March 2017 / Accepted: 10 March 2017 / Published online: 18 April 2017
© SSIEM and Springer-Verlag Berlin Heidelberg 2017

Abstract Fabry disease (FD) is a genetic X-linked, multisystemic, progressive lysosomal storage disorder (LSD). Depression has emerged as a disease complication, with prevalence estimates ranging from 15 to 62%. This is a pilot study examining the effects of psychological counseling for depression in FD on depression, adaptive functioning (AF), quality of life (QOL), and subjective pain experience. Telecounseling was also piloted, as it has beneficial effects in other chronic diseases which make in-person counseling problematic. Subjects completed 6 months of in-person or telecounseling with the same health psychologist, followed by 6 months without counseling. Self-report measures of depression, AF, QOL, and subjective pain were completed every 3 months. All subjects experienced improvements in depression, which were sustained during the follow-up period. Improvements in depression were correlated with improvements in mental health QOL and subjective pain severity, while improvements in mental health QOL were correlated with improvements in AF. While statistical comparison between counseling modes was not possible with the given sample size, relevant observations were noted. Recommendations for future research include replication of results with a

larger sample size and a longer counseling period. The use of video counseling may be beneficial. In conclusion, the present pilot study supports the efficacy of psychological treatment for depression in people with FD, highlighting the importance of having health psychologists housed in LSD treatment centers, rather than specialty psychology/psychiatry settings, to increase participation and decrease potential obstacles to access due to perceived stigma.

Introduction

Fabry disease (FD) is an X-linked lysosomal storage disorder (LSD) caused by mutations in the GLA gene, leading to deficiency of α-galactosidase A (α-gal A; EC 3.2.1.22) and resulting in storage of globotriaosylceramide (GL3) and related lipids in the lysosome. Incidence has historically been estimated at 1:40,000 male live births; however, recent data suggest as high as 1:3,000 (Hopkins et al. 2015), with a range of 1,250–117,000 worldwide (Laney et al. 2015). Symptoms and complications include acroparesthesia, fatigue, anhidrosis, angiokeratomas, GI symptoms, kidney failure, cardiovascular problems, and stroke (Desnick et al. 2003; MacDermot et al. 2001). Standard of care treatment is enzyme replacement therapy (ERT).

Depression is increasingly recognized as a complication of FD, with prevalence estimates ranging from 15 to 62% (Bolsover et al. 2014; Crosbie et al. 2009; Laney et al. 2013; Löhle et al. 2015; Schermuly et al. 2011; Wang et al. 2007). In the largest study ($n = 296$), Cole et al. (2007) reported that 46% of subjects met criteria for clinically significant depressive symptoms. Wang et al. (2007) found

Communicated by: Avihu Boneh, MD, PhD, FRACP

Electronic supplementary material: The online version of this chapter (doi:10.1007/8904_2017_21) contains supplementary material, which is available to authorized users.

N. Ali (✉) · D. Laney
Department of Human Genetics, Emory University School of Medicine, Atlanta, GA, USA
e-mail: Nadia.Ali@emory.edu

S. Gillespie
Department of Pediatrics, Emory University School of Medicine, Atlanta, GA, USA

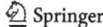

globally reduced quality of life (QOL) in FD women, with 62% reporting symptoms of depression and/or antidepressant treatment. While the most common factor associated with depression in FD is chronic pain (Bolsover et al. 2014; Cole et al. 2007), economic status, relationship status, and symptoms such as anhidrosis and acroparesthesia are also associated with depression and lower QOL (Cole et al. 2007; Gold et al. 2002). Löhle et al. (2015) found that antidepressants were more frequent among FD subjects than controls. Finally, FD does not follow gender norms, with males reporting greater depression than females (Cole et al. 2007; Sigmundsdottier et al. 2014).

While it is not understood whether depression is an organic symptom (Löhle et al. 2015), a result of Fabry-related cerebrovascular disease (Löhle et al. 2015), a reaction to coping with a chronic progressive condition (Campbell et al. 2003; Katon 2003), or a combination, it is clear that it needs to be taken seriously (Staretz-Chacham et al. 2010). Löhle et al. (2015) found that almost half of FD subjects reporting severe depression were undiagnosed and untreated. Few LSD centers integrate medical and psychological treatment, resulting in genetic counselors and nurses having to try to fill the psychosocial gap (Grosse et al. 2009; Hughes et al. 2006; Weber et al. 2012).

Untreated depression impacts self-management of chronic illness via negative effects on memory, energy, sense of well-being, and interpersonal interactions (Cole et al. 2007; Katon and Ciechanowski 2002). Consequences can include increased complication severity, pain intensity, and disability (Cole et al. 2007; Dersh et al. 2002; Katon 2003). Current FD treatment requires biweekly infusions, yet some patients are noncompliant despite the adverse health effects of missing infusions (West and LeMoine 2007).

While in-person psychological counseling is standard of care, telecounseling has become prevalent when in-person is not feasible. Research supports telecounseling for a range of concerns and populations (Stiles-Shields et al. 2014), including depression and post-traumatic stress disorder (Hilty et al. 2013; Jenkins-Guarnieri et al. 2015; Mohr et al. 2012), as well as chronic illnesses such as HIV/AIDS (Himelhoch et al. 2013), multiple sclerosis (Mohr et al. 2005, 2007), and breast cancer (Badger et al. 2005). In such populations, telecounseling can help with barriers to in-person counseling, including physical impairments, fatigue, transportation, lack of local specialized services, childcare, stigma, and lack of finances (Mohr et al. 2005; Hollon et al. 2002). When FD treatment at an infusion center is problematic, ERT is often administered via home health nursing agencies. For these patients, telecounseling may help them receive psychological treatment at home as well.

In summary, it is critical to assess depression in FD and expand standard of care to include mental health treatment where appropriate. The present study is a first step toward focused treatment of FD-associated depression. We hypothesize that counseling will improve depression and consequently adaptive functioning (AF), subjective pain severity, and overall QOL. Furthermore, we hypothesize that telecounseling will be as effective as in-person counseling.

Methods

Subjects were recruited through Emory's LSD Center from December 2010 through September 2013. Eligibility criteria included English-speaking individuals with FD ≥18 years old.

Subjects completed three self-report questionnaires: the Achenbach System of Empirically Based Assessment (ASEBA) Adult Self-Report (ASR) or Older Adult Self-Report (OASR), the Short Form 36-item Health Questionnaire (SF-36), and the Brief Pain Inventory (BPI). Subjects scoring within borderline-clinical to clinical ranges on the depression scale of the ASEBA were randomized into in-person counseling or telecounseling conditions. Any subject reporting suicidal ideation was excluded and referred to more intensive psychiatric care.

All subjects participated in counseling with the same health psychologist every 2 weeks for 6 months. Counseling was tailored to each subject's particular situation, utilizing a combination of cognitive behavioral tools (e.g., log-keeping for identification of triggers, journaling to identify patterns in cognition, goal-setting, and homework assignments pertaining to specific stressors) and insight-oriented techniques (e.g., exploration of themes in interpersonal relationships, understanding the influence of past circumstances and coping skills on present challenges, with a focus on increasing self-awareness and decreasing cognitive dissonance). Subjects repeated ASEBA ASR or OASR, SF-36, and BPI questionnaires at 3 and 6 months in counseling, as well as at post-counseling period (9 and 12 months), to measure sustainability of changes.

Measures

The ASEBA ASR is a reliable, validated measure of social-adaptive and psychological functioning in adults aged 18–59 and the OASR is for ages 60–90+ (Achenbach and Rescorla 2003). Norms represent the mix of ethnicities, socioeconomic status, urban–rural–suburban residency, and geography within the USA. Raw scores are converted to T-scores to permit comparisons with the general population. Scale scores are normed by gender and age and categorized as normal (<93rd percentile), borderline-clinical (93rd–97th percentiles), or clinical (>97th percentile). The ASEBA is used with a wide variety of medical

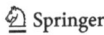

conditions, including cystic fibrosis, Fabry, Morquio, Turner, Williams, Angelman, and Prader–Willi syndromes (Achenbach and Rescorla 2003; Ali and Cagle 2015; Laney et al. 2010). For this study, the Depression scale and Mean Adaptive Functioning scale were used.

The BPI is a reliable, validated measure of pain severity and interference in daily life (Cleeland 2009). It yields mean Pain Severity (PS) and Pain Interference (PI) scores. PI scores consist of two dimensions (physical activity and affective) and measure how much subjects' pain interferes with general activity, mood, walking, normal work, relationships, sleep, and enjoyment of life. The BPI has been used with a variety of medical conditions, including Fabry and other LSDs (Ali and Cagle 2015; Cleeland 2009; Laney et al. 2010).

The SF-36 is a 36-item survey measuring QOL. Scores provide summary measurements of physical and mental well-being. Raw scores are converted to T-scores and norm-based. The SF-36 is a reliable, validated questionnaire (Maruish and DeRosa 2009; Maruish and Kosinski 2009) used with a variety of medical conditions, including Fabry and other LSDs (Ali and Cagle 2015; Hoffmann et al. 2005; Laney et al. 2010; Watt et al. 2010; Weinreb et al. 2007; Wilcox et al. 2008).

Data Analysis

ASEBA raw data was entered into assessment data manager (ADM) ASEBA scoring software. Subjects with T-scores in borderline-clinical and clinical ranges were considered symptomatic in depression and/or AF. Raw data from the SF-36 was entered into QualityMetric Health Outcomes Scoring Software 4.5, which utilizes T-scores to provide overall Physical Health Summary and Mental Health Summary scores. BPI raw data was scored according to the BPI User Guide (Cleeland 2009).

Statistical significance was evaluated at the 0.05 level. Data analyses were performed using SAS v9.4 (Cary, NC) and CRAN R v3.3 (Vienna, Austria). Patient demographics, treatment characteristics, and drug specifications were summarized using means and standard deviations for continuous variables and frequencies and percentages in discrete cases. Linear mixed regression models were utilized to gauge for change in measure score outcomes over patient follow-up (0, 3, 6, 9, and 12 months) in the full sample, adjusted for treatment type as a covariate. Residual errors for each modeled outcome were assessed for approximate normality via histograms, boxplots, and quantile–quantile probability plots. Post hoc t-tests, from the regression models, were employed for pairwise differences at follow-up timepoints relative to baseline and 6 months, respectively. Partial Pearson correlations, controlling for treatment type, considered linear associations between outcome measures in the full sample. Regression model estimates were plotted as model-based means and 95% confidence intervals; concurrently, raw data for each measure were plotted over patient follow-up, by treatment type, for visualization of individual and treatment trends. Finally, due to small sample size, statistically significant results noted in the linear regression models were further evaluated by nonparametric, exact Wilcoxon signed-rank tests, as a supplement. Being an exploratory study, no adjustments were made to p-values for multiple comparisons.

Results

Thirty-five FD adults were screened. Nineteen met inclusion criteria; however, two subjects enrolled in another study and two elected to withdraw before beginning counseling. A total of 15 subjects were thus randomly assigned (six to in-person counseling and nine to tele-counseling). However, five subjects (one from in-person counseling and four from telecounseling) withdrew prior to the 3-month timepoint. Withdrawal reasons included involuntary incarceration, disliking the telephone aspect of counseling, cessation of crisis period, and unknown. In total, ten subjects completed the study, five in each group. Due to the small number of subjects, and for purposes of statistical power, pilot analyses concentrated on all ten subjects without stratification.

Demographic characteristics are presented in Table 1. All subjects spoke English and reside in the USA. Ages ranged from 22 to 61 years.

Primary Results

Psychological Symptoms

Treatment-adjusted mean summary scores and standard errors by measure over time are presented in Table 2. Subjects experienced significant improvement in depression (Mean Difference: −7.5; t(df): −2.32(16.5); $p = 0.034$) over the 6-month counseling period (Table 3; Fig. 1). Improvements in other variables (i.e., adaptive function, QOL, and subjective pain levels) were noted, particularly with the SF-36-Mental scale, but statistically insignificant.

Subjects' improvement in depression was sustained over the post-counseling period; that is, depression scores at 9 months and 12 months remained significantly improved in comparison with scores at baseline (Mean Difference: −9.3 and −7.9; t(df): −3.55(17.5) and −2.49(15.9); $p = 0.002$ and $p = 0.024$, respectively). Moreover, depression scores at 9 and 12 months did *not* differ significantly from scores at counseling termination (Mean

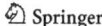

Table 1 Demographic characteristics: mean (standard deviation) or frequency (percentage)

Characteristic, N (%)	All participants, N = 10
Mean age (years), mean (SD)	42.1 (12.0)
Gender	
Women	8 (80%)
Men	2 (20%)
Race	
Caucasian-American	7 (70%)
African-American	1 (10%)
Asian-American	1 (10%)
Arab-American	1 (10%)
Education	
Less than HS	1 (10%)
Completed HS	3 (30%)
Completed college	4 (40%)
In or completed graduate school	2 (20%)
Employment	
Full-time worker	4 (40%)
Student	1 (10%)
Disabled	4 (40%)
None	1 (10%)
Marital status	
Married	6 (60%)
Divorced	2 (20%)
Widowed	1 (10%)
Single	1 (10%)
Medication for Fabry disease	
Agalsidase alpha	6 (60%)
Agalsidase beta	1 (10%)
AT1001	2 (20%)
None	1 (10%)
Use of psychiatric medicine	
Yes	4 (40%)
Intermittent	2 (20%)
No	4 (40%)

Difference: −1.8 and −0.4; t(df): −0.57(15.8) and −0.11 (17.7); $p = 0.576$ and $p = 0.914$, respectively) (Table 3). Due to small sample size, nonparametric testing of the depression scores was also conducted and are presented in Supplementary Table 2, demonstrating analogous results. Results in the supplementary table are presented as median differences, Wilcoxon signed-rank S-statistics, and p-values.

Finally, improvement in depression correlated significantly with both mental health QOL improvement ($r = 0.59$; $p < 0.001$) and pain severity improvement ($r = 0.35$; $p = 0.014$) (Supplementary Table 1). In addition, AF correlated with both physical ($r = -0.36$; $p = 0.010$)

and mental ($r = 0.33$; $p = 0.020$) components of QOL. Physical QOL was also correlated with the interference of pain in both physical ($r = -0.56$; $p < 0.001$) and mental ($r = -0.39$; $p = 0.006$) tasks (Supplementary Table 1).

Spaghetti plots by participants for each measure over time are presented in Supplementary Fig. 1.

Quality of Life

Subjects' scores on the SF-36 Physical Health component were not significantly different from the Mental Health component at any timepoint (Baseline: 37.7 versus 32.1, t (df): 1.2(18), $p = 0.246$; 3 months: 38.9 versus 37.1, t(df): 0.5(18), $p = 0.624$; 6 months: 36.7 versus 38.1, t(df): 0.3 (18), $p = 0.766$; 9 months: 34.4 versus 41; t(df): 1.58(18), $p = 0.132$; 12 months: 38.4 versus 37.8, t(df): 0.17(18), $p = 0.870$). However, scores on both components were significantly lower than the US mean score of 50 at all timepoints (p-values ranged from $p < 0.001$ to $p = 0.019$). Physical and Mental Health components were not significantly correlated (Baseline: $r = -0.43$, $p = 0.199$; 3 months: $r = -0.02$, $p = 0.962$; 6 months: $r = -0.37$, $p = 0.287$; 9 months: $r = 0.22$, $p = 0.532$; 12 months: $r = -0.38$, $p = 0.267$).

Pain

Pain Severity (PS) was significantly correlated with Pain Interference (PI) at 6 months ($r = 0.78$, $p = 0.004$), 9 months ($r = 0.71$, $p = 0.014$), and 12 months ($r = 0.63$, $p = 0.038$), but not baseline ($r = 0.49$, $p = 0.10$) or 3 months ($r = 0.58$, $p = 0.065$), albeit associations at these timepoints were moderate. Correlations observed were significant for both Physical Activity (6 months: $r = 0.70$, $p = 0.016$; 9 months: $r = 0.70$, $p = 0.017$; 12 months: $r = 0.65$, $p = 0.030$) and Affective (6 months: $r = 0.75$, $p = 0.007$; 9 months: $r = 0.69$, $p = 0.018$) dimensions, relative to Pain Severity.

Discussion

The present study may be considered a pilot study demonstrating the beneficial impact of psychological counseling for FD adults with depression. Benefits included lasting improvement in depression up to 6 months post-counseling, as well as associated improvements in QOL and subjective pain severity. Improvements in mental health QOL were associated with improvements in adaptive functioning.

While statistical analysis between telecounseling and in-person counseling conditions was not possible due to sample size, a number of observational comparisons were

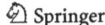

Table 2 Regression-adjusted summary scores and standard errors by measure over time

Measure, mean (SE)	0 months N = 10	3 months N = 10	6 months N = 10	9 months N = 10	12 months N = 10
Adjusted summaries					
Depression	75.0 (1.9)	67.2 (2.4)	67.5 (2.6)	65.7 (1.8)	67.1 (2.5)
Adaptive functioning	40.2 (2.6)	42.0 (3.2)	43.0 (2.5)	42.6 (2.3)	43.7 (3.0)
SF-36 – physical	37.7 (3.2)	38.9 (2.6)	36.7 (2.8)	34.4 (2.7)	38.4 (2.5)
SF-36 – mental	32.1 (3.4)	37.1 (2.5)	38.1 (3.7)	41.0 (3.2)	37.8 (2.6)
Pain severity score	3.1 (0.6)	4.0 (0.3)	3.2 (0.7)	3.1 (0.7)	2.9 (0.7)
Pain interference score	4.0 (1.0)	3.8 (0.6)	3.4 (0.8)	3.8 (0.9)	3.7 (0.9)
PIS – physical	3.8 (0.9)	3.5 (0.7)	3.3 (0.8)	3.4 (0.9)	3.6 (1.0)
PIS – mental	4.3 (1.1)	4.2 (0.7)	3.6 (0.9)	4.3 (1.0)	3.9 (0.9)

Table 3 Regression model-based tests comparing depression scores at 6, 9, and 12 months versus baseline and 6 months, adjusted for treatment arm[a]

Measure	6 months vs. baseline	9 months vs. baseline	12 months vs. baseline	9 months vs. 6 months	12 months vs. 6 months
Depression	−7.5; −2.32 (16.5); **0.034**	−9.3; −3.55 (17.5); **0.002**	−7.9; −2.49 (15.9); **0.024**	−1.8; −0.57 (15.8); 0.576	−0.4; −0.11 (17.7); 0.914

[a] Results presented as mean measure differences relative to baseline and 6 months, respectively; t(df); p-value

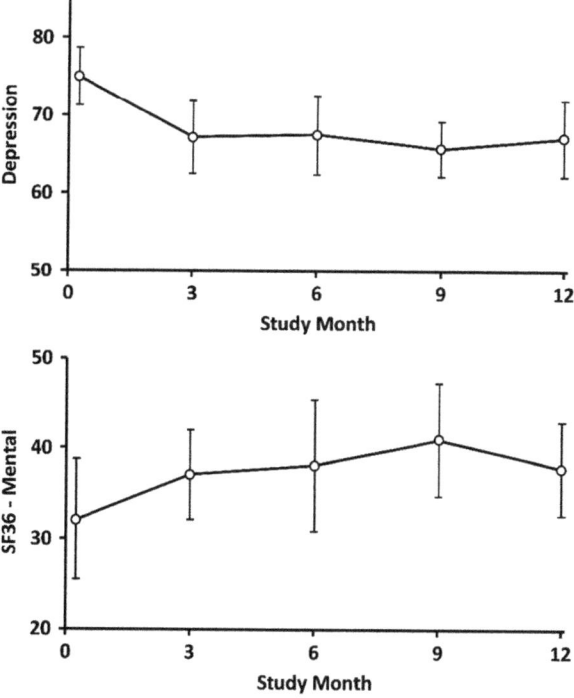

Fig. 1 Depression and SF-36-mental scores and 95% CI over follow-up visits, regression adjusted for treatment arm

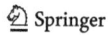

noted. First, telecounseling subjects tended to forget and/or reschedule sessions more often than in-person subjects. As counseling occurred on infusion days for the in-person group, these subjects may have had multiple reasons to remember appointments.

Second, most subjects who withdrew came from the telecounseling group. The only in-person withdrawal was involuntary due to incarceration. Subjects who withdrew did so within the first 3 months, one verbalizing that she disliked the telecounseling aspect. It is possible that others felt similarly, but did not say so. However, at least one remaining subject verbalized, "Having someone to talk to over the phone versus in-person allowed me to feel less nervous, able to be honest. When you are on the phone, you have to talk." This perspective mirrors Donnelly et al.'s (2000) findings with breast cancer patients that the familiar, informal nature of telephone contact led to more natural, "conversational" communications and subjects spoke more easily about intimate matters when they did not have to look the therapist in the face. Future research may differentiate characteristics regarding preference versus rejection of telecounseling more clearly.

From the psychologist's perspective, it was more difficult to interpret subjects' experiences without nonverbal cues or ascertain whether subjects were truly in a private place and/or engaged in other tasks rather than giving counseling their full attention. The use of video counseling may help in both regards and has been validated in populations such as PTSD (Germain et al. 2010) and geriatric depression (Choi et al. 2014a, b).

The finding that mental health QOL improvement was associated with AF improvement is important for several reasons. AF measures how effectively individuals cope with demands of everyday tasks and responsibilities. Laney et al. (2010) found AF deficits in FD patients to be higher than population norms, with poorer AF associated with greater depression, anxiety, antisocial personality, attention-deficit/hyperactivity and aggressive behavior. In comparison, only 10% of Morquio patients were observed to have mean AF deficits (Ali and Cagle 2015). While the reason for this difference is unclear, it suggests that Laney et al.'s results may be FD-specific, rather than due to chronic pain, LSD, or chronic disease in general. Our results, indicating counseling for depression in FD is associated with improved mental health QOL, which is associated with improved AF, suggest that AF may likewise be treatable via psychological counseling. While improvements in depression were not directly correlated with AF improvement, the small sample size may have prevented an effect from being realized, as counseling was not specifically for AF. Future research investigating psychological counseling for AF in FD is warranted.

Our finding that subjects' physical and mental health QOL were both significantly below the US mean is consistent with previous FD research (Arends et al. 2015; Crosbie et al. 2009; Gold et al. 2002; Watt et al. 2010; Wilcox et al. 2008). Subjects' improvement in QOL with counseling for depression lends credence to calls for integration of physical and psychological treatment in medical centers treating FD (Grosse et al. 2009; Hughes et al. 2006; Weber et al. 2012).

The bidirectional interaction between physical and psychological health is well-established. Biological evidence supports an overlap in the neural circuitry underlying physical and social pain (Eisenberger 2012). Multiple studies have found depression in patients with chronic illness to alter immune function, increase symptom burden and functional impairment, decrease adjustment to illness and coping skills, interfere with social functioning (e.g., irritability, withdrawal, and isolation behaviors), impede self-care and treatment compliance, and result in diminished use of the healthcare system, with resulting poorer overall medical outcomes and increased medical costs (Katon 2003; Katon and Ciechanowski 2002). On the other hand, good adjustment to illness is linked to increased attempts to gain control over one's health and better overall health outcomes. It is thus critical to monitor depressive symptoms associated with FD and expand standard of care to include mental health treatment when necessary. As reflected in one subject's feedback, "Counseling has made such a difference in learning to cope with chronic illness, family and work related issues. Life is very stressful in itself but learning comfortable coping tools has been the key to self-help."

The primary study limitation is the small sample size due to the rarity of FD. A larger sample may have revealed significant differences or correlations not currently detectable, as well as permitted statistical comparisons between telecounseling and in-person conditions. In addition, subjects who participated may have differed from those who chose not to participate. Ethnic variability also differed between groups; we cannot be sure of the cause or effect of this difference. Another necessary limitation was the exclusion of subjects expressing suicidality. While it was necessary to refer these subjects to more intensive psychiatric treatment, we acknowledge that doing so restricted the subject population to mild to moderate levels of depression. While some subjects were on antidepressant medications, these subjects had all been taking these medications for long periods of time prior to the commencement of the study, suggesting that something in addition to the medication contributed to the improvements observed over the relatively short-term period of the study. Finally, while measures chosen are all well-validated, reliable measures,

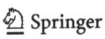

the use of self-report patient outcome measures may not have resulted in the same data as independent provider-rated outcome measures.

Recruitment was difficult due to several factors, including the rare nature of FD, a treatment shortage's impact on medical center visits, and the tendency for depressed patients to be noncompliant as a consequence of depression itself (Campbell et al. 2003; Deen et al. 2013; Mohr et al. 2005). Finally, the relatively short counseling period (i.e., biweekly for 6 months, totaling approximately 12 sessions) may have been a limiting factor. Two subjects mentioned this specifically – "The only thing I would change would be ending therapy in six months. I felt alone" and "My only concern was with the time period. Just as I started to notice that the counseling was helping, that part of the study ended."

Recommendations for future research include replication of results with a larger sample size and a longer counseling period and statistical comparison of in-person and tele-counseling. The use of video counseling may also increase efficacy.

In conclusion, this pilot study supports the efficacy and need for psychological treatment for depression in people with FD, highlighting the importance of having health psychologists housed in LSD treatment centers rather than specialty psychology/psychiatry settings, to increase participation and decrease potential obstacles to access due to perceived stigma (Grosse et al. 2009; Hughes et al. 2006; Weber et al. 2012; Campbell et al. 2003).

Acknowledgments The authors thank all the individuals with Fabry disease who participated in this study.

This study was supported by Shire Pharmaceuticals and by the National Center for Advancing Translational Sciences of the National Institutes of Health under Award Number UL1TR000454. The content is solely the responsibility of the authors and does not necessarily represent the official views of the National Institutes of Health.

One Sentence Take-Home Message

This study supports the efficacy of psychological counseling for depression in people with FD in improving mental health QOL.

Contributions of Individual Authors

Nadia Ali Ph.D. is responsible for conception and design of the research, data collection, data preparation and interpretation, and writing of the manuscript to be submitted for publication. She is the guarantor.

Dawn Laney M.S. is responsible for conception and design of research, securing grant funding, subject recruit-

ment, and reviewing the article before submission for publication.

Scott Gillespie M.S. is responsible for portions of the statistical analysis, assistance writing the data analysis section of the manuscript, and construction of figures and tables.

Conflicts of Interest

Nadia Ali Ph.D. has received research support from Genzyme, Shire, BioMarin, and Pfizer, as well as lecturers' honoraria from Genzyme, BioMarin, and Amicus. These activities are monitored and are in compliance with the conflict of interest policies at Emory University.

Dawn Laney M.S. consults for Genzyme and Shire and is a study coordinator in clinical trials sponsored by Genzyme, Amicus, and Protalix. She has also received research funding from Alexion, Amicus, Genzyme, Pfizer, Retrophin, Shire, and Synageva. These activities are monitored and are in compliance with the conflict of interest policies at Emory University.

Scott Gillespie M.S. has no conflicts of interest to declare.

Funding Source

Shire Pharmaceuticals.

The author(s) confirm independence from the sponsors; the content of the article has not been influenced by the sponsors.

Informed Consent

All procedures followed were in accordance with the ethical standards of the responsible committee on human experimentation (institutional and national) and with the Helsinki Declaration of 1975, as revised in 2000 (5). Informed consent was obtained from all patients for being included in the study. Emory University IRB reviewed and approved the conduct of this study.

References

Achenbach TM, Rescorla LA (2003) Manual for the ASEBA adult forms and profiles. University of Vermont, Research Center for Children, Youth, and Families, Burlington. www.aseba.org

Ali N, Cagle S (2015) Psychological health in adults with Morquio syndrome. JIMD Rep 20:87–93

Arends M, Hollak CEM, Biegstraaten M (2015) Quality of life in patients with Fabry disease: a systemic review of the literature. Orphanet J Rare Dis 10:77

Badger T, Segrin C, Meek P, Lopez AM, Bonham E, Sieger A (2005) Telephone interpersonal counseling with women with breast

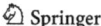

cancer – symptom management and quality of life. Oncol Nurs Forum 32(2):273–279

Bolsover FE, Murphy E, Cipolotti L, Werring DJ, Lachmann RH (2014) Cognitive dysfunction and depression in Fabry disease: a systemic review. J Inherit Metab Dis 37(2):177–187

Campbell LC, Clauw DJ, Keefe FJ (2003) Persistent pain and depression: a biopsychosocial perspective. Biol Psychiatry 54(3):399–409

Choi NG, Hegel MT, Marti CN, Narinucci ML, Sirrianni L, Bruce ML (2014a) Telehealth problem-solving therapy for depressed low-income homebound older adults – acceptance and preliminary efficacy. Am J Geriatr Psychiat 22(3):263–271

Choi NG, Wilson NL, Sirrianni L, Marinucci ML, Hegel MT (2014b) Acceptance of home-based telehealth problem-solving therapy for depressed, low-income homebound older adults: qualitative interviews with the participants and aging-service case managers. Gerontologist 54(4):704–713

Cleeland CS (2009) The brief pain inventory user guide. MD Anderson Cancer Center, Houston

Cole AL, Lee PJ, Hughes DA, Deegan PB, Waldeck S, Lachmann RH (2007) Depression in adults with Fabry disease: a common and underdiagnosed problem. J Inherit Metab Dis 30:943–951

Crosbie TW, Packman W, Packman S (2009) Psychological aspects of patients with Fabry disease. J Inherit Metab Dis 32:745–753

Deen T, Fortney J, Schroeder G (2013) Patient acceptance, initiation, and engagement in telepsychotherapy in primary care. Psychiatr Serv 64(4):380–384

Dersh J, Polatin PB, Gatchel RJ (2002) Chronic pain and psychopathology: research findings and theoretical considerations. Psychosom Med 64:773–786

Desnick RJ, Brady R, Barranger J, Collins AJ, Germain DP et al (2003) Fabry disease, an under-recognized multisystemic disorder: expert recommendations for diagnosis, management, and enzyme replacement therapy. Ann Intern Med 138:338–346

Donnelly JM, Kornblith AB, Fleishman S, Zuckerman E, Raptis G et al (2000) A pilot study of interpersonal psychotherapy by telephone with cancer patients and their partners. Psycho-Oncol 9:44–56

Eisenberger NI (2012) The pain of social disconnection: examining the shared neural underpinnings of physical and social pain. Nat Rev Neurosci 13(6):421–434

Germain V, Marchand A, Bouchard S, Guay S, Drouin M (2010) Assessment of the therapeutic alliance in face-to-face or videoconference treatment for posttraumatic stress disorder. Cyberpsychol Behav Soc Netw 13(1):29–35

Gold KF, Pastores GM, Botteman MF et al (2002) Quality of life of patients with Fabry disease. Qual Life Res 11:317–327

Grosse SD, Schechter MS, Kulkarni R et al (2009) Models of comprehensive multidisciplinary care for individuals in the United States with genetic disorders. Pediatrics 123:407–412

Hilty DM, Ferrer DC, Parish MB, Johnston B, Callahan EJ, Yellowlees PM (2013) The effectiveness of telemental health: a 2013 review. Telemed J E Health 19(6):444–454

Himelhoch S, Medoff D, Maxfield J et al (2013) Telephone based cognitive behavioral therapy targeting major depression among urban dwelling, low income people living with HIV/AIDS: results of a randomized controlled trial. AIDS Behav 17:2756–2764

Hoffmann B, Garcia de Lorenzo A, Mehta A et al (2005) Effects of enzyme replacement therapy on pain and health related quality of life in patients with Fabry disease: data from FOS (Fabry Outcome Survey). J Med Genet 42:247–252

Hollon S, Munoz RF, Barlow DH, Beardslee WR, Bell CC, Bernal G et al (2002) Psychosocial intervention development for the prevention and treatment of depression: promoting innovation and increasing access. Biol Psychiatry 52:610–630

Hopkins PV, Campbell C, Klug T et al (2015) Lysosomal storage disorder screening implementation: finding from the first six months of full population pilot testing in Missouri. J Pediatr 166(1):172–177

Hughes DA, Evans S, Milligan A et al (2006) A multidisciplinary approach to the care of patients with Fabry disease. In: Mehta A, Beck M, Sunder-Plassmann G (eds) Fabry disease: perspectives from 5 years of FOS. Oxford PharmaGenesis, Oxford

Jenkins-Guarnieri MA, Pruitt LD, Luxton DD, Johnson K (2015) Patient perceptions of telemental health: systematic review of direct comparisons to in-person psychotherapeutic treatments. Telemed J E Health 21(8):1–9

Katon WJ (2003) Clinical and health services relationships between major depression, depressive symptoms, and general medical illness. Biol Psychiatry 54:216–226

Katon W, Ciechanowski P (2002) Impact of major depression on chronic medical illness. J Psychosom Res 53:859–863

Laney DA, Gruskin DJ, Fernhoff PM et al (2010) Social-adaptive and psychological functioning of patients affected by Fabry disease. J Inherit Metab Dis 33(Suppl 3):S73–S81

Laney DA, Bennett RL, Clarke V, Fox A, Hopkin RJ, Johnson J et al (2013) Fabry disease practice guidelines: recommendations of the National Society of Genetic Counselors. J Genet Couns 22:555–564

Laney DA, Peck DS, Atherton AM et al (2015) Fabry disease in infancy and early childhood: a systematic literature review. Genet Med 17(5):323–330

Löhle M, Hughes D, Milligan A et al (2015) Clinical prodromes of neurodegeneration in Anderson-Fabry disease. Neurology 84:1454–1464

MacDermot KD, Holmes A, Miners AH (2001) Anderson-Fabry disease: clinical manifestations and impact of disease in a cohort of 60 obligate carrier females. J Med Genet 38:769–775

Maruish ME, DeRosa MA (2009) A guide to the integration of certified Short Form survey scoring and data quality evaluation capabilities. QualityMetric Incorporated, Lincoln

Maruish ME, Kosinski M (2009) A guide to the development of certified short form interpretation and reporting capabilities. QualityMetric Incorporated, Lincoln

Mohr DC, Hart SL, Julian L, Catledge C et al (2005) Telephone-administered psychotherapy for depression. Arch Gen Psychiatry 62:1007–1014

Mohr DC, Hart SL, Vella L (2007) Reduction in disability in a randomized controlled trial of telephone-administered cognitive-behavioral therapy. Health Psychol 26(5):554–563

Mohr DC, Ho JH, Duffecy J, Reifler D et al (2012) Effect of telephone-administered vs in-person cognitive behavioral therapy on adherence to therapy and depression outcomes among primary care patients. JAMA 307(21):2278–2285

Schermuly I, Muller MJ, Muller KM, Albrecht J, Keller I et al (2011) Neuropsychiatric symptoms and brain structural alterations in Fabry disease. Eur J Neurol 18:357–353

Sigmundsdottier L, Tchan MC, Knopman AA, Menzies GC et al (2014) Cognitive and psychological functioning in Fabry disease. Arch Clin Neuropsychol 29:642–650

Staretz-Chacham O, Choi JH, Wakabayashi K et al (2010) Psychiatric and behavioral manifestations of lysosomal storage disorders. Am J Med Genet B Neuropsychiatr Genet 153B:1253–1265

Stiles-Shields C, Kwasny MJ, Cai X, Mohr DC (2014) Therapeutic alliance in face-to-face and telephone-administered cognitive behavioral therapy. J Consult Clin Psychol 82:349–354

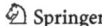

Wang RY, Lelis A, Mirocha J, Wilcox WR (2007) Heterozygous Fabry women are not just carriers, but have a significant burden of disease and impaired quality of life. Genet Med 9(1):34–45

Watt T, Burlina AP, Cazzorla C et al (2010) Agalsidase beta treatment is associated with improved quality of life in patients with Fabry disease: findings from the Fabry Registry. Genet Med 12:703–712

Weber SL, Segal S, Packman W (2012) Inborn errors of metabolism: psychosocial challenges and proposed family systems model of intervention. Mol Genet Metab 105:537–541

Weinreb N, Barranger J, Packman S et al (2007) Imiglucerase (Cerezyme) improves quality of life in patients with skeletal manifestations of Gaucher disease. Clin Genet 71(6):576–588

West M, LeMoine K (2007) Withdrawal of enzyme replacement therapy in Fabry disease: indirect evidence of treatment benefit? Mol Genet Metab 92(4):32

Wilcox WR, Oliveira JP, Hopkin RJ et al (2008) Females with Fabry disease frequently have major organ involvement: lessons from the Fabry Registry. Mol Genet Metab 93:112–128

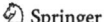

JIMD Reports
DOI 10.1007/8904_2017_25

RESEARCH REPORT

Mutations in *GMPPB* Presenting with Pseudometabolic Myopathy

Chiara Panicucci · Chiara Fiorillo · Francesca Moro ·
Guja Astrea · Giacomo Brisca · Federica Trucco ·
Marina Pedemonte · Paola Lanteri · Lucia Sciarretta ·
Carlo Minetti · Filippo M. Santorelli · Claudio Bruno

Received: 06 January 2017 / Revised: 03 April 2017 / Accepted: 04 April 2017 / Published online: 30 April 2017
© SSIEM and Springer-Verlag Berlin Heidelberg 2017

Abstract Mutations in the guanosine diphosphate mannose (GDP-mannose) pyrophosphorylase B (*GMPPB*) gene encoding a key enzyme of the glycosylation pathway have been described in families with congenital (CMD) and limb girdle (LGMD) muscular dystrophy with reduced alpha-dystroglycan (α-DG) at muscle biopsy.

Patients typically display a combined phenotype of muscular dystrophy, brain malformations, and generalized epilepsy. However, a wide spectrum of clinical severity has been described ranging from classical CMD presentation to children with mild, yet progressive LGMD with or without intellectual disability. Cardiac involvement, including a long QT interval and left ventricular dilatation, has also been described in four cases.

Two missense mutations in *GMPPB* gene, one novel and one already reported, have been identified in a 21-year-old man presenting with elevated CK (38,650 UI/L; normal values <150 UI/L) without overt muscle weakness. Major complaints included limb myalgia, exercise intolerance, and several episodes of myoglobinuria consistent with a form of metabolic myopathy. Muscle biopsy showed only minimal alterations, whereas a marked reduction of glycosylated α-DG was evident.

This case further expands the phenotypic spectrum of *GMPPB* mutations and highlights the importance of exhaustive molecular characterization of patients with reduced glycosylation of α-DG at muscle biopsy.

Communicated by: Jaak Jaeken, Em. Professor of Paediatrics

"Chiara Panicucci" and "Chiara Fiorillo" equally contributed to this work.

C. Panicucci · G. Brisca · C. Bruno (✉)
Center of Myology and Neurodegenerative Disorders, Department of Neuroscience and Rehabilitation, Istituto Giannina Gaslini, Genoa, Italy
e-mail: claudio2246@gmail.com

C. Panicucci · C. Fiorillo · C. Minetti
University of Genoa, Genoa, Italy

C. Fiorillo · F. Trucco · M. Pedemonte · C. Minetti
Pediatric Neurology Unit, Istituto Giannina Gaslini, Genoa, Italy

F. Moro · G. Astrea · F. M. Santorelli
Neuromuscular and Molecular Medicine Unit, IRCCS Stella Maris Foundation, Pisa, Italy

P. Lanteri · L. Sciarretta
Infantile Neuropsychiatry Unit, Department of Neuroscience and Rehabilitation, Istituto Giannina Gaslini, Genoa, Italy

Introduction

Congenital muscular dystrophies with hypoglycosylation of alpha-dystroglycan (α-DG) are a heterogeneous group of disorders of varying severity often associated with brain and eye defects in addition to muscular dystrophy.

Seventeen genes have been implicated in defective α-DG glycosylation, including proteins with putative or uncertain glycosyltransferase function such as POMT1, POMT2, POMGNT1, LARGE, GTD2, B4GAT1, B3GALNT2; one protein implicated in a glycan phosphorylation SGK-196; proteins involved in mannose, dolichol, and ribitol metabolism such as GMPPB, DPM1, DPM2, DPM3, DOLK, and other largely uncharacterized genes such as *FKTN*, *FKRP*, *ISPD*, and *TMEM5* (Bouchet-Seraphin et al. 2015; Gerin et al. 2016). Allelic mutations in some of these genes have been also linked to milder limb-girdle muscular dystrophy phenotype such as LGMD2I (*FKRP*), LGMD2K (*POMT1*), LGMD2M (*FKTN*), LGMD2N (*POMT2*), LGMD2O (*POMGnT1*), and LGMD2U (*ISPD*) (Gerin et al. 2016).

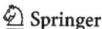

Among them mutations in *FKRP* are quite common, leading to at least 10% of all LGMD (Nigro and Savarese 2014).

The most recently added gene to the list is the guanosine diphosphate mannose pyro phosphorylase B (*GMPPB*) gene. The guanosine diphosphate mannose pyro phosphorylase B encodes an enzyme involved in α-DG glycosylation; in particular, it catalyzes the formation of GDP-mannose, which is required for O-mannosylation of proteins. As expected, a defect of GMPPB results in hypoglycosylation of α-DG in human cells and animal models (Carss et al. 2013; Raphael et al. 2014; Cabrera-Serrano et al. 2015; Bharucha-Goebel et al. 2015; Belaya et al. 2015; Jensen et al. 2015; Oestergaard et al. 2016; Montagnese et al. 2016; Gerin et al. 2016).

GMPPB causative variants have been described so far in 49 cases with a spectrum of clinical phenotypes ranging from forms with structural brain and eye anomalies (OMIM615350) to forms with a limb-girdle phenotype (LGMD2T – OMIM 615352). In particular a predominant mild LGMD phenotype associated with *GMPPB* mutation is described in 29 patients.

Recently also congenital myasthenic syndromes have been reported with patients with *GMPPB* mutation (CMS-GMPPB) and EMG myasthenic patterns have been observed in LGMD-GMPPB patients (Belaya et al. 2015; Montagnese et al. 2016).

Generalized epilepsy has been described in 12 patients (Carss et al. 2013; Raphael et al. 2014; Cabrera-Serrano et al. 2015; Bharucha-Goebel et al. 2015; Belaya et al. 2015; Jensen et al. 2015) and evidence of cardiorespiratory involvement including a long QT interval, sino-atrial block, wandering atrial pacemaker, bicuspid aortic valve, and left ventricular dilatation in seven patients (Carss et al. 2013; Cabrera-Serrano et al. 2015; Jensen et al. 2015). Furthermore, mild to severe mental retardation is reported in 24 patients (Carss et al. 2013; Raphael et al. 2014; Cabrera-Serrano et al. 2015; Bharucha-Goebel et al. 2015; Belaya et al. 2015; Jensen et al. 2015; Oestergaard et al. 2016) and ophthalmologic features as cataracts or strabismus have been described in 9 cases (Carss et al. 2013; Bharucha-Goebel et al. 2015; Jensen et al. 2015). Cerebellar hypoplasia at brain MRI is reported in 6 patients with severe mental retardation and CMD phenotype (Carss et al. 2013 and Jensen et al. 2015). Muscle MRI data from 11 patients have been published so far (Bharucha-Goebel et al. 2015; Belaya et al. 2015; Oestergaard et al. 2016; Montagnese et al. 2016). In one of the most recent papers (Oestergaard et al. 2016) the authors defined a specific muscle MRI pattern associated with LGMD-GMPPB

patients which preferentially involves paraspinal and hamstring muscles.

Here we describe a further case harboring two missense mutations in *GMPPB* and presenting mild features consistent with a metabolic muscle disorder. We also provide a summary of the main characteristics observed in previously described LGMD-GMPPB patients (Table 1).

Case Report

The propositus, a 23-year-old man, is the second child of healthy unrelated parents. He was born at term after uneventful pregnancy and normal delivery. Psychomotor development was reported normal. At 6 years, he showed generalized epileptic seizures and he was put on valproate therapy which was continued until 12 years of age despite no further epileptic manifestations. Last EEG, performed at the age of 14 years, was normal.

At the age of 15 years he came to observation for a first episode of acute rhabdomyolysis after moderate exercise. CK level at the time was 38,650 UI/L and myoglobinuria was reported. Subsequently, serum CK level dropped to 2,100 UI/L in follow-up measurements and remained elevated thereafter, despite substantial abstinence from physical activity.

On neurological examination there was no motor defect. We only observed mild calf hypertrophy and flat feet. Wechsler Adult Intelligence Scale – Revised (WAIS-R) showed a generalized moderate mental retardation (verbal IQ 48; performance IQ 45).

Respiratory muscles function was spared with normal spirometry. ECG documented short PR interval and prolonged QRS, with occasional delta waves, indicating Wolf–Parkinson–White syndrome. Echocardiography was normal for chambers dimensions, morphology, and ejection fraction. At 23 years the patient underwent ablation of the abnormal electrical pathway by radiofrequency catheter.

At 16 years, a muscle biopsy revealed moderate fiber size variability with several hypotrophic fibers (Fig. 1a) and increased staining for acid phosphatase (Fig. 1b). Most hypotrophic fibers were type I. The immunofluorescence study of sarcolemmal proteins revealed a significant reduction of α-DG binding (Fig. 1c–e). Western blot analysis with anti-IIH6 antibody showed a 15% reduction of α-DG levels compared to the control (Fig. 1f). Serum CK level was 1,062 UI/L at the time of the muscle biopsy.

Muscle MRI at 21 years revealed a moderate increase in T1 hyperintensity in posterior tights muscles, hamstrings, and very mild involvement of soleus (Fig. 1g). A subsequent

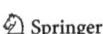

Table 1 Summary of the main clinical, lab and genetic features of previously described GMPPB patient with LGMD phenotype

	Sex	Origin	Onset	Muscular symptoms	Neurological features	Cardiorespiratory features	Ophthalmologic features	CK level (UI/L)	Neurophysiology	Brain MRI findings	Muscle MRI findings	Genetical findings	Reference
P1	F	Indian	Birth	Not shown	Mild intellectual disability / Epilepsy	None	None	4,500	Not performed	No structural abnormality	Not performed	c.64C>T c.1000G>A	Carss et al. (2013)
P2	M	English	4 years	Mild exercise intolerance	None	None	None	3,000	Not performed	Not performed	Not performed	c.79G>C c.988G>A	Carss et al. (2013)
P3	M	Egyptian	2.5 years	Mild lower limb weakness	Mild intellectual disability / Epilepsy	Wandering atrial pacemaker / Cardiomyopathy / Respiratory insufficiency	Cataract, nystagmus	5,200	Not performed	No structural abnormality	Not performed	c.553C>T c.553C>T	Carss et al. (2013)
P4	M	Australian	15 years	Difficulties in running / Exercises intolerance / Calves hypertrophy	Behavioral problems	None	None	5,000	Myopathic EMG	Not performed	Not performed	c.79G>C c.95C>T	Cabrera-Serrano et al. (2015)
P5	M	Australian	26 years	Lower limb weakness / Calves hypertrophy	None	Right bundle branch block	None	3,600–17,000	Not performed	Not performed	Not performed	c.79G>C c.95C>T	Cabrera-Serrano et al. (2015)
P6	F	Italian	28 years	Upper and lower limb weakness / Calves hypertrophy	None	Respiratory insufficiency at 70 years	None	Not shown	Myopathic EMG	Not performed	Not performed	c.79G>C c.797G>A	Cabrera-Serrano et al. (2015)
P7	M	Italian	35 years	Upper and lower limb weakness / Calves hypertrophy	None	Sino-atrial block	None	1,000	Not performed	Not performed	Not performed	c.79G>C c.797G>A	Cabrera-Serrano et al. (2015)
P8	M	Caucasian	22 years	Upper and lower limb weakness	Learning difficulties / Autism	None	None	1,400	Not performed	Not performed	Not performed	c.79G>C c.1036C>A	Cabrera-Serrano et al. (2015)
P9	M	Caucasian	22 years	Upper and lower limb weakness	Learning difficulties	None	None	1,400	Not performed	Not performed	Not performed	c.79G>C c.1036C>A	Cabrera-Serrano et al. (2015)
P10	M	Unknown	13 years	Recurrent rhabdomyolysis	Rolandic epilepsy	None	None	700 baseline 35,000 in crises	Not performed	Not performed	Not performed	c.860G>A c.95C>T	Cabrera-Serrano et al. (2015)
P11	M	Unknown	12 years	Mild exercise intolerance / Upper and lower limb weakness (MRC4/5) / Calves hypertrophy	Intellectual disability (IQ 49) / ADHD / Epilepsy (6 years)	None	Cataract (severe)	18,000	Myopathic EMG	Bilateral cortical thinning	Normal muscle bulk, mild T1 signal increase	c.79G>C c.790C>T	Bharucha-Goebel et al. (2015)
P12	F	Unknown	12 years	Muscle pain / Upper and lower limb weakness (MRC4/5) / Calves hypertrophy	Intellectual disability (IQ 58)	None	Cataract (mild)	15,000	Myopathic EMG	Normal	Normal muscle bulk, mild T1 signal increase	c.79G>C c.790C>T	Bharucha-Goebel et al. (2015)
P13	F	Unknown	13 years	Mild exercise intolerance / Upper and lower limb weakness (MRC4/5) / Calves hypertrophy	Mild intellectual disability (IQ 81)	Not investigated	Cataract (mild)	3,000	Not performed	Not performed	Normal muscle bulk, mild T1 signal increase	c.79G>C c.790C>T	Bharucha-Goebel et al. (2015)

(continued)

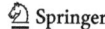

Table 1 (continued)

	Sex	Origin	Onset	Muscular symptoms	Neurological features	Cardiorespiratory features	Ophthalmologic features	CK level (UI/L)	Neurophysiology	Brain MRI findings	Muscle MRI findings	Genetical findings	Reference
P14	F	Caucasian	15 years	Episodes of generalized sudden weakness	None	Not investigated	None	3,000	Myopathic EMG decrement on repetitive nerve stimulation	Not performed	Not performed	c.559C>T c.578T>C	Belaya et al. (2015)
P15	M	Caucasian	2.5 years	Upper and lower limb weakness	Mild intellectual disability	Not investigated	None	3,000	Myopathic EMG Increase in jitter + block on SFEMG	Not performed	Not performed	c.656T>C c.860G>A	Belaya et al. (2015)
P16	M	Caucasian	2 years	Upper and lower limb weakness	Moderate intellectual disability	Not investigated	None	2,832	Increase in jitter	Not performed	Not performed	c.656T>C c.860G>A	Belaya et al. (2015)
P17	F	Asian	2.5 years	Upper and lower limb weakness	Moderate intellectual disability	Not investigated	None	2,500	Normal	Not performed	Not performed	c.64C>T c.1000G>A	Belaya et al. (2015)
P18	M	Unknown	17 years	Muscle weakness	Epilepsy None	Ischemic heart disease	None	1,331	Not performed	Not performed	Not performed	c.79G>C c.1069G>A	Jensen et al. (2015)
P19	M	Unknown	17 years	Mild exercise intolerance with myalgias and myoglobinuria	None	None	None	7,250 baseline 52,000 in crises	Not performed	Not performed	Not performed	c.79G>C c.1069G>A	Jensen et al. (2015)
P20	M	Unknown	15 years	Muscle weakness	None	None	None	3,693	Not performed	Not performed	Not performed	c.79G>C c.760G>A	Jensen et al. (2015)
P21	M	Unknown	23 years	Incidental hyperCKemia Myoglobinuria	None	Atrio-ventricular block (1st degree)	None	5,900	Not performed	Not performed	Not performed	c.79G>C c.402+1G>A	Jensen et al. (2015)
P22	F	Unknown	5 years	Muscle weakness	Moderate intellectual disability	Moderate restrictive lung disease	None	7,112	Not performed	Not performed	Not performed	c.721C>T c.1034T>C	Jensen et al. (2015)
P23	M	Caucasian	15 years	Difficulties in running	None	FVC 59%	None	2,390	Myopathic EMG decrement on repetitive nerve stimulation	Normal	Severe T1 signal increase in paraspinal (MS 4) and hamstring (MS 4) muscles	c.79G>C c.859C>T	Oestergaard et al. (2016)
P24	F	Caucasian	30 years	Difficulties in climbing stairs	None	FVC 66%	None	1,520	Not performed	Normal	Severe T1 signal increase in paraspinal (MS 4) and hamstring (MS 4) muscles	c.79G>C c.859C>T	Oestergaard et al. (2016)
P25	F	Caucasian	12 years	Difficulties in running	None	FVC 76%	None	1,604	Myopathic EMG decrement on repetitive nerve stimulation	Normal	Mild T1 signal increase in paraspinal (MS 3) and hamstring (MS 2) muscles	c.464G>A c.1039_1043 dup	Oestergaard et al. (2016)
P26	F	Caucasian	18 years	Exercise intolerance	MMSE 27/30	None	None	1,200	Myopathic EMG decrement on repetitive nerve stimulation	Normal	Mild T1 signal increase in paraspinal (MS 2) and hamstring (MS 2) muscles	c.79G>C c.760G>A	Oestergaard et al. (2016)
P27	M	Caucasian	5 years	Walked at 5 years	Not reported	FVC 61%	None	1,327	Not performed	Normal	Not performed	c.79G>C c.859C>T	Oestergaard et al. (2016)
P28	M	Caucasian	25 years	Difficulties in walking	MMSE 28/30	FVC 43% Ejection fraction 48%	None	619	Myopathic EMG decrement on repetitive nerve stimulation	Normal	Not performed	c.902C>G c.1069G>A	Oestergaard et al. (2016)

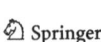

P29	M	Unknown	8 years	Calves hypertrophy Myoglobinuria Action tremor	None	None	None	3,000 baseline 25,000 in crises	Myopathic EMG normal repetitive nerve stimulation	Normal	Mild edematous changes of soleus muscles	c.79G>C c.859C>T	Montagnese et al. (2016)
P30	M	Caucasian	15 years	Mild exercise intolerance with myalgias and myoglobinuria	Moderate intellectual disability (IQ 45)	WPW syndrome	None	2,000 baseline 38,000 in crises	Myopathic EMG normal repetitive nerve stimulation	Slight pericerebellar subarachnoid space enlargement	Mild T1 signal increase in hamstring muscles (MS2)	c.79G>C c.943C>A	This report

MRC Medical Research Council evaluation of strength, *MMSE* Mini-Mental State Examination, *WPW* Wolf-Parkinson-White, *FVC* forced vital capacity, *SFEMG* single fibre EMG, *MS* Mercuri scale

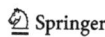

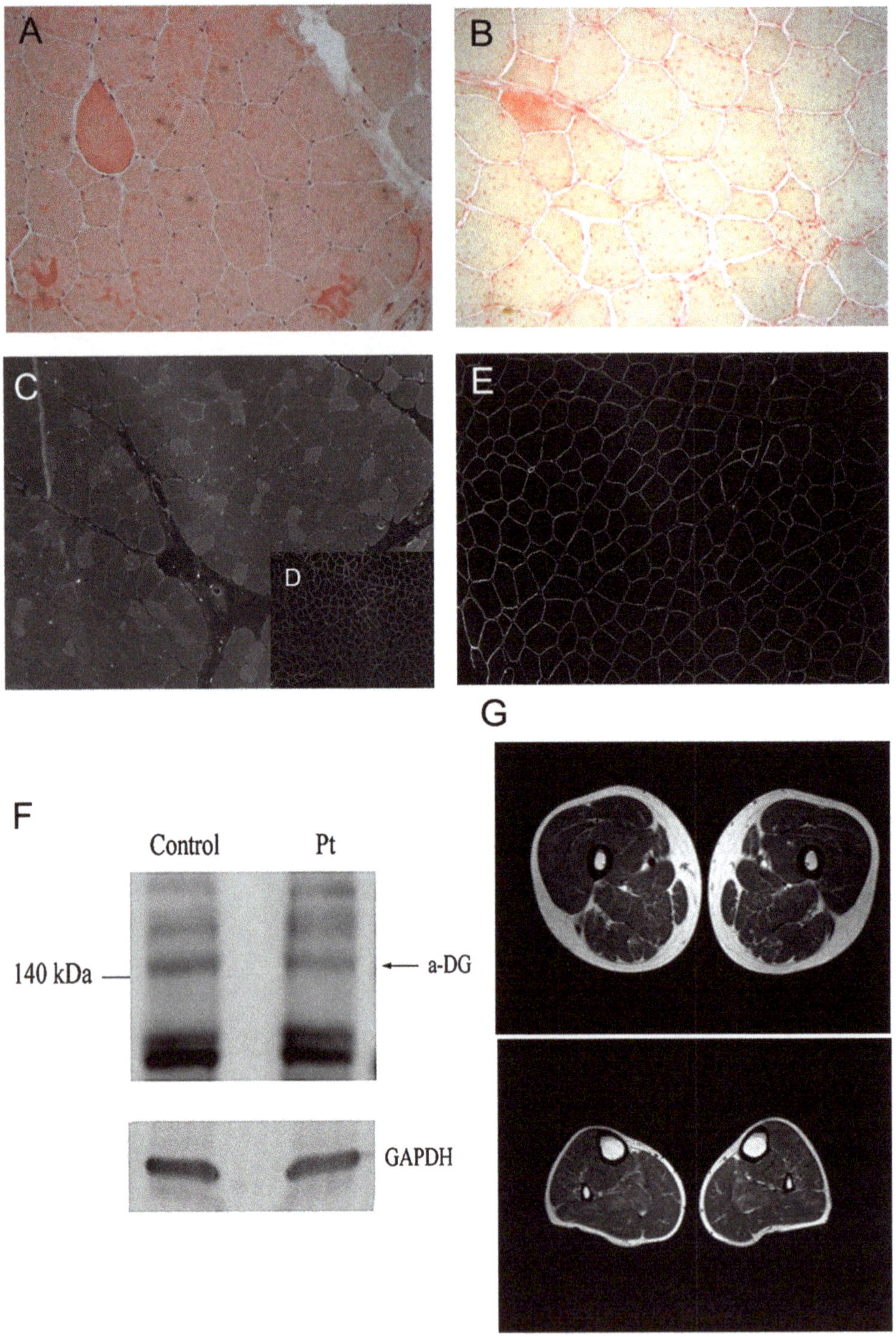

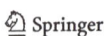

Fig. 1 (**A**, **B**) Histology of skeletal muscle from the patient. Hematoxylin eosin staining showed moderate fiber size variability with several hypotrophic fibers and some hypercontracted fibers (**A**). The staining for acid phosphatase was increased (**B**). (**C**–**E**) Immunofluorescence with IIH6C4 antibody showing profound reduction of immunodetectable glycosylated α–DG (**C**) in comparison to control muscle stained with the same antibody (**D**). In (**E**) immunofluorescence for caveolin-3, showing normal protein expression. (**F**) Western blotting showed an expected band of 140 kDa with a 15% reduction in glycosylated α-DG compared to control. Anti-α-Dystroglycan, clone IIH6, monoclonal antibody (Millipore, Temecula, CA) was used at 1:100 dilution, according to manufacturer's instruction. GADPH expression is used as control for protein loading. Band intensities were evaluated by densitometry using the ImageQuant 350 system (Amersham Biosciences). (**G**) Muscle MRI performed at 21 years disclosed a moderate fatty infiltration in muscles of the posterior thigh (adductor magnus hamstrings, and partially sartorius) and minimal fatty infiltration of soleus muscle at leg level

muscle MRI at 23 years showed a stable picture of muscle involvement (data not shown).

Brain MRI performed at the age of 23 years did not reveal definite abnormalities except for slight pericerebellar subarachnoid space enlargement.

Latest neurological examination at the age of 23 years showed minimal muscle strength reduction (MRC 4) of pelvic girdle muscles. Deep tendon reflexes were reduced in all limbs. Pseudo-hypertrophy of calves and quadriceps, and a mild scoliotic curve were evident. In view of the recent work by Belaya et al. (2015) reporting myasthenic features in GMPPB patients, we performed repetitive nerve stimulation of the left median nerve which did not reveal any pathological findings.

Genetic analysis of the most common form of alpha-dystroglycanopathy with milder phenotype did not show pathogenic mutations in *FKRP, POMT-1, POMT-2, LARGE, FKTN,* and *ISPD*. This case was included in a group of undiagnosed muscular dystrophy patients to be analyzed by Dystroplex, an extended NGS testing panel able to investigate, in a single tube, the coding regions of 93 genes linked to CMDs, LGMDs, and related diseases. We identified a c.79G>C (p.D27H) on the maternal allele and a c.943C>A (p. G315S) on the paternal allele. The latter variant is novel and affects a highly conserved residue and it is considered damaging on Polyphen prediction software.

Mutation c.79G>C (p.D27H) has been previously reported in 19 cases presenting with LGMD phenotype, whereas it has never been described in association with CMD.

Discussion

Exercise myalgia and rhabdomyolysis are commonly suggestive of an underlying metabolic condition, such as a glycogen storage disorder, fatty acid oxidation disorder, or mitochondrial cytopathy. However, there are anecdotal reports of pseudometabolic dominant clinical manifestations of defined genetic muscular diseases.

Pseudometabolic symptoms have been frequently reported in patients with dystrophin gene mutations with neither fixed muscle weakness nor calf hypertrophy. Patients harbored in-frame deletion, rarely missense mutations. In some cases immunohistochemical analysis demonstrated normal dystrophin staining for antibodies against the COOH-terminus and rod domain, and dystrophin western blot analysis confirmed normal dystrophin quantity (Minetti et al. 1993; Figarella-Branger et al. 1997; Veerapandiyan et al. 2010; Liewluck et al. 2015). Exertional myalgia and rhabdomyolysis may also be a presenting feature in female carriers of X-linked dystrophinopathies (Itagaki et al. 1993).

In 2007 Nguyen et al., retrospectively examining clinical data from 40 patients with dysferlin deficiency associated with LGMD2B phenotype, found that four patients had distal leg painful swelling without any weakness or atrophy (Nguyen et al. 2007).

Likewise two different series of patients with genetically confirmed LGMD2I due to mutations in the *FKRP* gene displayed a high incidence (26–37%) of pseudometabolic presentation (Mathews et al. 2011; Lindberg et al. 2012). Most of these patients were homozygous for the common p. L276I mutation and exercise-induced muscle cramps and myoglobinuria were the only presenting symptom occurring before the onset of muscle weakness.

There are a few reports on pseudometabolic presentation in patients affected by LGMD1C, LGMD2A, LGMD2C, LGMD2D, LGMD2E, and LGMD2L (Aboumousa et al. 2008; Penisson-Besnier et al. 1998; Pena et al. 2010; Ceravolo et al. 2014; Mongini et al. 2002; Cagliani et al. 2001; Lahoria et al. 2014; Quinlivan and Jungbluth 2012).

So far among patients carrying disease-related variants in *GMMPB* only four other similar cases have been reported, three of them carrying the same c.79G>C p.D27H variant presented by our patient (Jensen et al. 2015; Montagnese et al. 2016). One child showed also a severe muscle impairment beside the metabolic presentation, whereas the other patients showed exclusively post-exercise rhabdomyolysis with myoglobinuria.

Some hypotheses have been postulated to account for the pseudometabolic presentation in patients with muscular dystrophies, even if the mechanisms involved are not completely clear. It is widely accepted that deficiency of one or more components of the dystrophin associated protein complex (DPC) leads to an increased membrane susceptibility to contraction-induced damage. This process has been largely studied in *mdx* mice, the animal model of DMD, and seems to be due to a structural weakness of the sarcolemma and to impaired homeostasis resulting from increased membrane permeability to Ca2+ and Na+ (Gillis 1999; Allen 2004). It has been suggested that the cyto-skeletal disarrangement, due to dystrophin defect, can induce abnormalities of enzyme complexes organization and function, which in turn alter the control of energy metabolism in the muscle cells (Even et al. 1994). Finally it has been demonstrated that the level of sarcolemmal damage is directly correlated with the magnitude of mechanical stress (Petrof et al. 1993).

Thus it is possible that the milder end of the muscular dystrophies is able to a heavier workload, and as a consequence is more prone to rhabdomyolysis. The present patient, carrying two mutations in *GMPPB* gene, presented with exertional myalgias and myoglobinuria. In addition muscle biopsy showed increased acid phosphatase staining which can be considered the hallmark of several metabolic

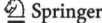

myopathies such as glycogenosis type 2. The muscle MRI disclosed a mild involvement of the hamstring muscles that has recently been defined as a common finding in LGMD2T (Oestergaard et al. 2016). Interestingly, our patient, carrying the c. c.79G>C p.D27H substitution which shows an allelic frequency of 32.7% among LGMD-GMPPB patients, confirms the mild muscular phenotype associated with this *GMPPB* variant (Carss et al. 2013; Oestergaard et al. 2016; Montagnese et al. 2016). It has also been suggested that the p.D27H retains more functional activity than other mutants found in more severe phenotypes as demonstrated by C2C12 myoblasts transfection experiments (Carss et al. 2013). Aside from the predominant pseudometabolic presentation, the boy suffered from epileptic seizures in childhood which remitted in adolescence. These did not differ from common idiopathic benign epilepsy of childhood. There is limited information on the type and severity of epilepsia in GMPPB. Drug resistant epileptic seizure has been mostly associated with more severe phenotypes but to our knowledge no cases have been described with benign epilepsy. The boy also suffered from WPW syndrome and underwent ablation of the abnormal electrical pathway. WPW has a prevalence of 1/450, and it has never been described in association with mutations in *GMMPB*. Taking all this into account a possible concomitant presentation of both epilepsy and WPW cannot be excluded. Albeit a decremental result at repetitive nerve stimulation (RNS) and good response to pyridostigmine have been reported in some GMPPB patients (Belaya et al. 2015), we have not pursued this therapy because of lack of suggestive RNS findings and in fear of low compliance from the patient who suffers from moderate mental retardation.

In conclusion, our case extends the number of patients with pseudometabolic presentation of limb girdle muscle dystrophies. An alpha-dystroglycanopathy should be considered in the differential diagnosis of the most common metabolic myopathies in order to provide a correct genetic counseling and long-term surveillance.

Acknowledgments The authors wish to thank the patient and his family for the collaboration, and Paolo Broda and Annagloria Incontrera for technical assistance.

Take Home Message

In this report we highlight the importance of considering an α-DG glycosylation defect when a pseudometabolic phenotype occurs.

Compliance With Ethics Guidelines

Conflict of Interest

Chiara Panicucci, Chiara Fiorillo, Francesca Moro, Guja Astrea, Giacomo Brisca, Federica Trucco, Marina Pedemonte, Paola Lanteri, Lucia Sciarretta, Carlo Minetti, Filippo M. Santorelli, and Claudio Bruno declare that they have no conflict of interest.

Informed Consent

All procedures followed were in accordance with the ethical standards of the responsible committee on human experimentation (institutional and national) and with the Helsinki Declaration of 1975, as revised in 2000. Informed consent was obtained from all patients for being included in the study.

Author Contributions

Study concept and design: Panicucci, Fiorillo, Bruno.

Acquisition of data: Panicucci, Fiorillo, Moro, Astrea, Trucco, Lanteri, Sciarretta.

Analysis and interpretation of data: Panicucci, Fiorillo, Brisca, Pedemonte, Lanteri, Sciarretta, Bruno.

Drafting of the manuscript: Panicucci, Fiorillo, Pedemonte, Bruno.

Critical revision of the manuscript for important intellectual content: Fiorillo, Minetti, Santorelli, Bruno.

Obtained funding: Santorelli, Bruno.

Administrative, technical, and material support: Santorelli, Bruno.

Study supervision: Fiorillo, Bruno.

References

Aboumousa A, Hoogendijk J, Charlton R, Barresi R, Herrmann R, Voit T, Hudson J, Roberts M, Hilton-Jones D, Eagle M, Bushby K, Straub V (2008) Caveolinopathy-new mutations and additional symptoms. Neuromuscul Disord 18(7):572–578

Allen DG (2004) Brief review skeletal muscle function: role of ionic changes in fatigue, damage and disease. Clin Exp Pharmacol Physiol 31:485–493

Belaya K, Rodríguez Cruz P, Liu W, Maxwell S, McGowan S, Farrugia M, Petty R, Walls T, Sedghi M, Basiri K, Yue W, Sarkozy A, Bertoli M, Pitt M, Kennett R, Schaefer A, Bushby K, Parton M, Lochmuller H, Palace J, Muntoni F, Beeson D (2015) Mutations in GMPPB cause congenital myasthenic syndrome and

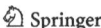

bridge myasthenic disorders with dystroglycanopathies. Brain 138:2493–2504

Bharucha-Goebel DX, Neil E, Donkervoort S, Dastgir J, Wiggs E, Winder TL, Moore SA, Iannaccone ST, Bönnemann CG (2015) Intrafamilial variability in GMPPB-associated dystroglycanopathy: broadening of the phenotype. Neurology 84(14):1495–1497

Bouchet-Seraphin C, Vuillaumier-Barrot S, Seta N (2015) Dystroglycanopathies: about numerous genes involved in glycosylation of one single glycoprotein. J Neuromuscul Dis 2:27–38

Cabrera-Serrano M, Ghaoui R, Ravenscroft G, Johnsen RD, Davis MR, Corbett A, Reddel S, Sue CM, Liang C, Waddell LB, Kaur S, Lek M, North KN, MacArthur DG, Lamont PJ, Clarke NF, Laing NG (2015) Expanding the phenotype of GMPPB mutations. Brain 138(Pt 4):836–844

Cagliani R, Comi GP, Tancredi L, Sironi M, Fortunato F, Giorda R, Bardoni A, Moggio M, Prelle A, Bresolin N, Scarlato G (2001) Primary beta-sarcoglycanopathy manifesting as recurrent exercise-induced myoglobinuria. Neuromuscul Disord 11:389–394

Carss KJ, Stevens E, Foley AR, Cirak S, Riemersma M, Torelli S, Hoischen A, Willer T, van Scherpenzeel M, Moore SA, Messina S, Bertini E, Bönnemann CG, Abdenur JE, Grosmann CM, Kesari A, Punetha J, Quinlivan R, Waddell LB, Young HK, Wraige E, Yau S, Brodd L, Feng L, Sewry C, MacArthur DG, North KN, Hoffman E, Stemple DL, Hurles ME, van Bokhoven H, Campbell KP, Lefeber DJ, Lin YY, Muntoni F, UK10K Consortium (2013) Mutations in GDP-mannose pyrophosphorylase B cause congenital and limb-girdle muscular dystrophies associated with hypoglycosylation of α-dystroglycan. Am J Hum Genet 93(1):29–41

Ceravolo F, Messina S, Rodolico C, Strisciuglio P, Concolino D (2014) Myoglobinuria as first clinical sign of a primary alpha-sarcoglycanopathy. Eur J Pediatr 173:239–242

Even PC, Decrouy A, Chinet A (1994) Defective regulation of energy metabolism in mdx-mouse skeletal muscles. Biochem J 304:649–654

Figarella-Branger D, Baeta Machado AM, Putzu GA, Malzac P, Voelckel MA, Pellissier JF (1997) Exertional rhabdomyolysis and exercise intolerance revealing dystrophinopathies. Acta Neuropathol 94:48–53

Gerin I, Ury B, Breloy I et al (2016) ISPD produces CDP-ribitol used by FKTN and FKRP to transfer ribitol phosphate onto alpha-dystroglycan. Nat Commun 7:11534. doi:10.1038/ncomms1153

Gillis JM (1999) Understanding dystrophinopathies: an inventory of the structural and functional consequences of the absence of dystrophin in muscles of the mdx mouse. J Muscle Res Cell Motil 20:605–625

Itagaki Y, Saida K, Nishitani H, Matsuo M, Nishio H (1993) Manifesting carriers of duchenne muscular dystrophy over two generations. Rinsho Shinkeigaku 33:377–381

Jensen B, Willer T, Saade D, Cox M, Mozaffar T, Scavina M, Stefans V, Winder T, Campbell K, Moore S, Mathews K (2015) GMPPB-associated dystroglycanopathy: emerging common variants with phenotype correlation. Hum Mutat 36:1159–1163

Lahoria R, Winder TL, Lui J, Al-Owain MA, Milone M (2014) Novel ANO5 homozygous microdeletion causing myalgia and unprovoked rhabdomyolysis in an Arabic man. Muscle Nerve 50(4):610–613

Liewluck T, Tian X, Wong LJ, Pestronk A (2015) Dystrophinopathy mimicking metabolic myopathies. Neuromuscul Disord 25:653–657

Lindberg C, Sixt C, Oldfors A (2012) Episodes of exercise-induced dark urine and myalgia in LGMD 2I. Acta Neurol Scand 125:285–287

Mathews KD, Stephan CM, Laubenthal K, Winder TL, Michele DE, Moore SA, Campbell KP (2011) Myoglobinuria and muscle pain are common in patients with limb-girdle muscular dystrophy 2I. Neurology 76(2):194–195

Minetti C, Tanji K, Chang HW et al (1993) Dystrophinopathy in two young boys with exercise-induced cramps and myoglobinuria. Eur J Pediatr 152:848–851

Mongini T, Doriguzzi C, Bosone I, Chiadò-Piat L, Hoffman EP, Palmucci L (2002) Alpha-sarcoglycan deficiency featuring exercise intolerance and myoglobinuria. Neuropediatrics 33:109–111

Montagnese F, Klupp E, Karampinos DC, Biskup S, Gläser D, Kirschke JS, Schoser B (2016) Two patients with GMPPB mutation: the overlapping phenotypes of limb-girdle myasthenic syndrome and LGMD2T dystroglycanopathy. Muscle Nerve. doi:10.1002/mus.25485

Nguyen K, Bassez G, Krahn M, Bernard R, Laforet P, Labelle V et al (2007) Phenotypic study in 40 patients with dysferlin gene mutations: high frequency of atypical phenotypes. Arch Neurol 64:1176–1182

Nigro V, Savarese M (2014) Genetic basis of limb-girdle muscular dystrophies: the 2014 update. Acta Myol 33(1):1–12

Oestergaard ST, Stojkovic T, Dahlqvist JR, Bouchet-Seraphin C, Nectoux J, Leturcq F, Cossée M, Solè G, Thomsen C, Krag TO, Vissing J (2016) Muscle involvement in limb-girdle muscular dystrophy with GMPPB deficiency (LGMD2T). Neurol Genet 2(6):e112

Pena L, Kim K, Charrow J (2010) Episodic myoglobinuria in a primary gamma-sarcoglycanopathy. Neuromuscul Disord 20:337–339

Penisson-Besnier I, Richard I, Dubas F, Beckmann JS, Fardeau M (1998) Pseudometabolic expression and phenotypic variability of calpain deficiency in two siblings. Muscle Nerve 21:1078–1080

Petrof BJ, Shrager JB, Stedman HH, Kelly AM, Sweeney HL (1993) Dystrophin protects the sarcolemma from stresses developed during muscle contraction. Proc Natl Acad Sci U S A 90(8):3710–3714

Quinlivan R, Jungbluth H (2012) Myopathic causes of exercise intolerance with rhabdomyolysis. Dev Med Child Neurol 54(10):886–891

Raphael AR, Couthouis J, Sakamuri S, Siskind C, Vogel H, Day JW, Gitler AD (2014) Congenital muscular dystrophy and generalized epilepsy caused by GMPPB mutations. Brain Res 1575:66–71

Veerapandiyan A, Shashi V, Jiang YH, Gallentine WB, Schoch K, Smith EC (2010) Pseudometabolic presentation of dystrophinopathy due to a missense mutation. Muscle Nerve 42:975–979

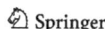

JIMD Reports
DOI 10.1007/8904_2017_27

RESEARCH REPORT

Heterogeneous Phenotypes in Lipid Storage Myopathy Due to *ETFDH* Gene Mutations

Corrado Angelini · Daniela Tavian · Sara Missaglia

Received: 23 January 2017 / Revised: 06 April 2017 / Accepted: 10 April 2017 / Published online: 30 April 2017
© SSIEM and Springer-Verlag Berlin Heidelberg 2017

Abstract We present six novel patients affected by lipid storage myopathy (LSM) presenting mutations in the *ETFDH* gene. Although the diagnosis of multiple acyl-coenzyme-A dehydrogenase deficiency (MADD) in adult life is difficult, it is rewarding because of the possibility of treating patients with carnitine or riboflavin, leading to a full recovery. In our patients, a combination of precipitating risk factors including previous anorexia, alcoholism, poor nutrition, and pregnancy contributed to a metabolic critical condition that precipitated the catabolic state.

In the present series of cases, five novel mutations have been identified in the *ETFDH* gene. We propose clinical guidelines to screen patients with LSM due to different defects, in order to obtain a fast diagnosis and offer appropriate treatment. In such patients, early diagnosis and treatment as well as avoiding risk factors are part of clinical management.

Specific biochemical studies are indicated to identify the type of LSM, such as level of free carnitine and acyl-carnitines and studies or organic acidemia. Indeed, when a patient is biochemically diagnosed with secondary carnitine deficiency, a follow-up with appropriate clinical-molecular protocol and genetic analysis is important to establish the final diagnosis, since riboflavin can be supplemented with benefit if riboflavin-responsive MADD is present. In muscle biopsies, increased lipophagy associated with p62-positive aggregates was observed. The clinical improvement can be attributed to the removal of an autophagic block, which appears to be reversible in this LSM.

Introduction

Lipid Storage Myopathies (LSMs) are a heterogeneous group of disorders of lipid metabolism characterized by impaired oxidation of fatty acids (FAs). LSM can arise from different defects in lipid metabolism (carnitine transport, beta-oxidation, and endogenous triglyceride catabolism); almost all associated with dys-metabolism of FAs and their derivatives (Liang and Nishino 2011).

Primary Systemic Carnitine Deficiency (SCD, MIM# 212140) is due to a defect in the plasma membrane high-affinity carnitine transporter (OCTN2, encoded by *SLC22A5* gene), causing systemic carnitine depletion.

In Multiple Acyl-coenzyme-A Dehydrogenase Deficiency (MADD, MIM# 231680), symptoms and age at onset are highly variable and characterized by recurrent episodes of lethargy, vomiting, hypoglycaemia, metabolic acidosis, and hepatomegaly, often preceded by a metabolic stress. Muscle involvement, myalgia, weakness, and LSM may occur. MADD is also known as "*glutaric aciduria type II*", because it results in large excretion of glutaric, lactic, ethyl-malonic, butyric, isobutyric, 2-methyl-butyric, and isovaleric acids. The organic aciduria in late-onset MADD patients is often intermittent and evident during illness or catabolic stress.

A clinical improvement of MADD myopathy following riboflavin supplementation has been observed in patients affected by either the infantile-severe, the adult, or the late-onset myopathic form. Most late-onset cases are characterized by a secondary carnitine-deficient LSM. MADD can be caused by mutations in three different genes (*ETFA*,

Communicated by: Avihu Boneh, MD, PhD, FRACP

C. Angelini (✉)
IRCCS San Camillo Hospital, Venice, Italy
e-mail: corrado.angelini@unipd.it

D. Tavian · S. Missaglia
CRIBENS – Laboratory of Cellular Biochemistry and Molecular Biology, Catholic University, Milan, Italy

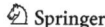

ETFB, and *ETFDH*) which are involved in the electron transfer in the mitochondrial respiratory chain. In most MADD patients, the disease is caused by mutations in the *ETFDH* gene (MIM # 231675), encoding the ETF dehydrogenase enzyme protein.

We present six patients affected by a carnitine-deficient LSM, with novel mutations in the *ETFDH* gene.

Methods

Patients

We investigated six patients from four families affected with a carnitine/riboflavin-responsive form of LSM. The diagnosis was based on characteristic muscle pathology features, low levels of plasma/muscle carnitine, high levels of acyl-carnitines, and glutaric acidemia.

Clinical re-evaluation was done during follow-up, including neuromuscular examinations, muscle MRI or CT imaging, and blood sample collection for genetic analysis.

Muscle Biopsy

Informed consent was obtained from all patients for undergoing muscle biopsy as part of the diagnostic procedure. Muscle biopsies were used for histopathological evaluation, following a panel of routine histochemical and histoenzymatic stains, and for ultrastructural analysis.

Biochemical Analysis

Carnitine and its fractions (acyl-carnitines) were extracted from muscle and plasma and their levels were determined using a standardized radiochemical method. Organic acids profile was investigated by mass spectrometry. Mitochondrial respiratory chain enzymes activity (OX-PHOS) was measured by a standard spectrophotometric method.

Genetic Analysis

Genomic DNA was extracted from blood sample using a standard method, and used for sequencing analysis of all exons and their flanking regions of the *ETFDH* gene.

Case Reports

Patient 1

This woman was hospitalized at age 36 years for psychiatric disturbances, alcoholism, and poor nutrition. She referred muscle pain in the upper limbs and weakness in the lower limbs with difficulty walking. She was unable to rise from the floor without assistance, had lost body weight over previous months, had difficulty walking and rising from a chair, and was unable to climb stairs. She was inadequately nourished, and her weakness had progressed steadily. She presented temporal lobe epilepsy, CK = 868 U/L, myopathic EMG, and had a subacute onset of carnitine-deficient LSM. Plasma acyl-carnitines and urinary organic acids profiles indicated an increased acyl-carnitine level. There was glutaric aciduria type II (ethyl-malonic acid = 70.5 nMol/mol creatinine, normal values 0.1–17.9). Muscle biopsy revealed LSM and low muscle carnitine levels (11% of controls). Mitochondrial enzyme activities were decreased in muscle after normalization to citrate synthase: NADH-dehydrogenase = 286.2 (normal values 391–663 nmol/min non-collagen protein), NADH-Cytochrome C reductase = 17.5 (n.v. 21.3–86.9), and Succinate Cytochrome C reductase = 4.35 (n.v.5.8–19.1). Treatment with a low-fat, high-protein diet and 4 g/day L-carnitine (because of secondary muscle carnitine deficiency with elevated acyl-carnitines) produced some improvement; however, only riboflavin supplementation (200 mg/day) produced marked improvement.

At age 45 years, she presented a crisis after an *ab-ingestis* pneumonia with septic shock, metabolic acidosis, dysphagia, and respiratory insufficiency, which required tracheostomy and assisted ventilation. On neurological examination, she had waddling gait, diffuse hypotonia, and weakness in lower limbs and hand grip. She slowly improved with carnitine, riboflavin, and carbamazepine.

Patient 2

This woman at age 38 years had a subacute onset of weakness of upper and lower girdle muscles, neck flexors, and respiratory muscles and became virtually quadriplegic and respirator-dependent. CK was 2,277 U/L, and a polymyositis was suspected. A steroid therapy was therefore tried for a short period of time while the patient was in intensive care unit. EMG was myopathic. A first muscle biopsy showed carnitine-deficient LSM with abnormal palmitate oxidation, which demonstrates a block of beta-oxidation. Treatment with a low-fat, high-protein diet, medium-chain triglyceride (MCT) oil supplementation, and 4 g/day of L-carnitine (because of muscle carnitine deficiency with increased acyl-carnitines and low palmitate beta-oxidation) produced some improvement and normalization of carnitine in plasma and muscle in a post-treatment muscle biopsy, which showed a decreased amount of lipid droplets but atrophic fibres. Riboflavin supplements (200 mg/day) produced improvement, preventing further metabolic crises. A muscle CT scan was recently repeated and showed only a mild muscle atrophy in both legs.

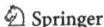

Patient 3

This 23-year-old woman presented extremely thin and weak muscles of undetermined cause. She complained of progressive arm, trunk, and lower limb weakness and exercise intolerance, developed myalgias, and had difficulty riding a bike or raising arms. One year later she had a thrombosis of inferior cava vein, recurrent episodes of hypoglycaemia (31 mg/dL), vomiting, conspicuous (10 kg) body weight loss, high CK (15,000 U/L), and diffuse myalgias. She became virtually quadriplegic due to nutritional deficiency (body weight was 48 kg) and had to be fed by nasogastric tube. On neurological examination, she presented a waddling gait, was able to go from a lying to sitting position only with the help of hands, could neither raise her arms in horizontal position nor raise legs from bed, and had a proximal muscle hypotrophy, winging scapulae, and distal leg hypotrophy. Manual muscle test by the MRC scale showed severe weakness of head flexors, deltoid, biceps, triceps, and arms extra-rotators, and of lower girdle muscles, especially of iliopsoas, tibialis anterior, peroneus, and EDL. On spirometry, a moderate restrictive deficiency

was found. Brain MRI was normal, and muscle MRI revealed oedema and marked atrophy of upper girdle, thigh, and leg muscles (Fig. 1).

Muscle biopsy showed the features of LSM (Fig. 2). We found a reduction of total muscle carnitine (4.34, n.v. 10.5–29.5), total plasma carnitine (6.77 mMol/L, n.v. 36.2–72.9), and free plasma carnitine (3.34 nMol/mL, n.v. 27.6–61.9) (Table 1). Plasma acyl-carnitines profile by mass spectroscopy was normal. Because of carnitine deficiency in muscle and plasma, she was treated simultaneously with riboflavin (200 mg/day) and L-carnitine (2 g/day) both orally and by infusion; with this treatment she could have her nasogastric tube removed and then, when she was able to walk, only by oral therapy. She gained body weight and muscle strength.

Patient 4

This is the older sister of patient 3. She was a 28-year-old, overweight woman, had experienced progressive lower limb weakness and myalgias for 4 years, and exercise intolerance, intermittent hypoglycaemic episodes, and

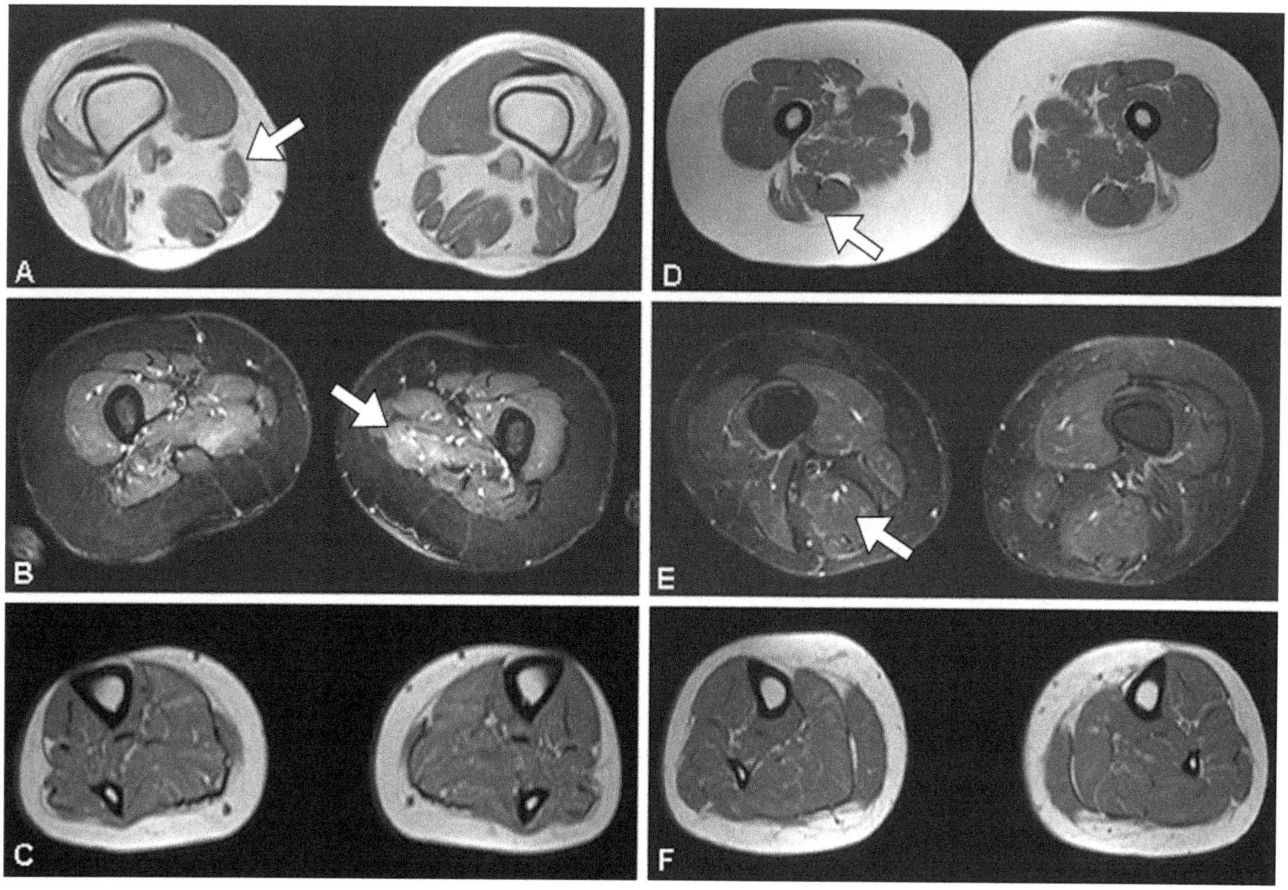

![Muscle MRI imaging of patients 3 and 4]

Fig. 1 Muscle MRI imaging in patient 3 (**a**, **b**, **c**) and patient 4 (**d**, **e**, **f**) using T1 sequences (**a**, **d**, **c**, **f**) and STIR sequences (**b**, **e**). Note atrophy of the thigh muscles (**a**, **b**) and in the leg muscles (**c**) in patient 3, while thigh muscles (**d**, **e**) and leg muscles (**f**) in patient 4 are not atrophic. Note hyper-intense signal in STIR sequences at the thigh level (**b**, **e**) due to myo-oedema

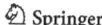

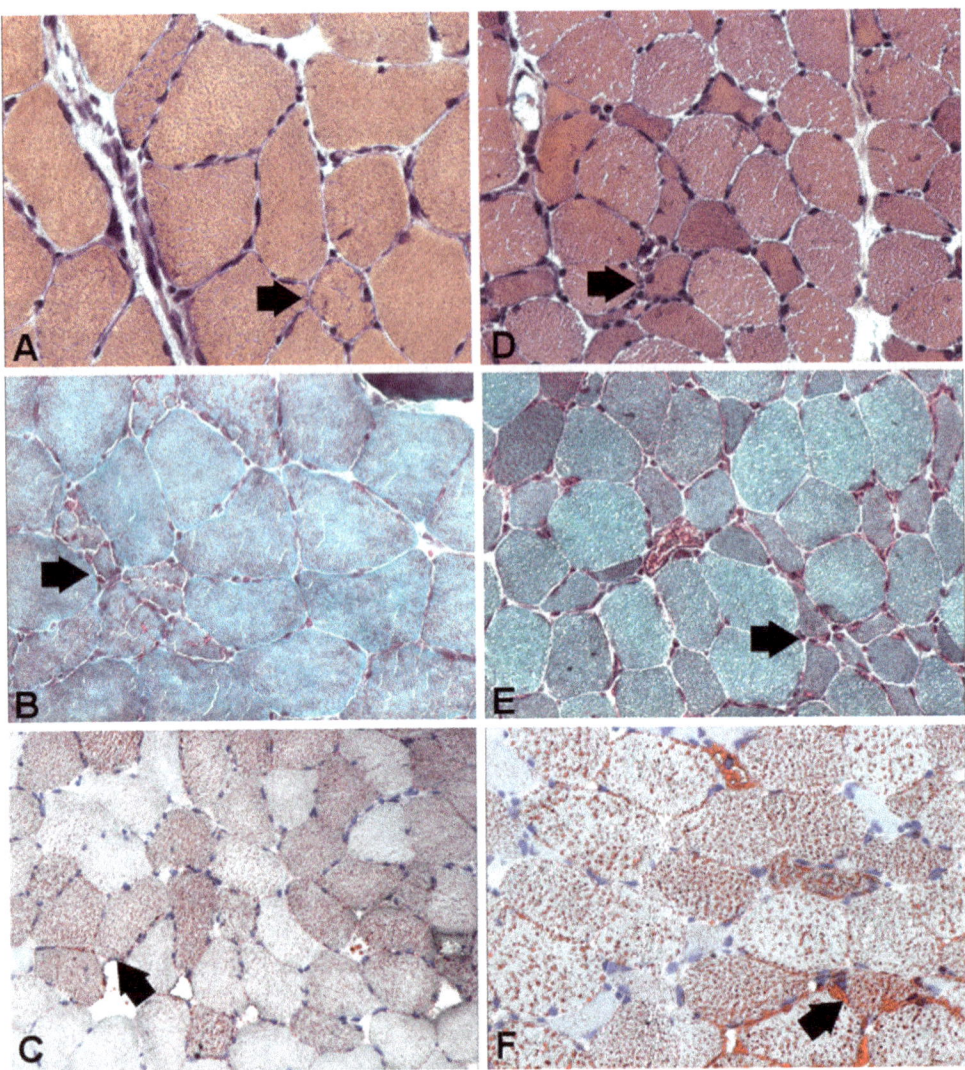

Fig. 2 Muscle biopsy morphology in patient 3 (**a**, **b**, **c**) and patient 4 (**d**, **e**, **f**) stained for hematoxylin-eosin (**a**, **d**), Gomori trichrome (**b**, **e**), and Oil-Red-O (**c**, **f**). Note that in patient 3 there is lipid storage and fibre size variability, whereas in patient 4 there are many atrophic fibres (**d**, **e**) and lipid storage (**f**). The atrophy is likely due to a prolonged steroid treatment

increased CK (11,000 U/L). She was misdiagnosed with polymyositis, and treated with IVIg, steroids (caused a cushingoid syndrome), methotrexate, and mycophenolate mofetil (Cell-cept) without benefit. On neurological examination, she had slow gait, kyphoscoliosis, slight weakness of head flexors, deltoid, arm extra-rotators, and iliopsoas muscles. CK was 188 U/L. Spirometry was normal. On abdominal ultrasound, a slight hepatomegaly was found. Muscle biopsy showed an LSM (Fig. 2). Muscle carnitine level was reduced (1.77, n.v. 10.5–29.5). Plasma acyl-carnitine profile was normal. She was started treatment with riboflavin (200 mg/day) and L-carnitine (2 g/day) and regained muscle strength.

Patient 5

This 16-year-old girl presented an acute post-partum carnitine deficiency syndrome, previously described (Angelini et al. 1978). She had generalized muscle weakness after the delivery, and, 2 months later had neck and limb muscle weakness, and myalgia and was unable to chew or lift arms and was quadriplegic. On muscle biopsy, there was an LSM, with low plasma and muscle carnitine levels (10%). She slowly recovered following a low-fat diet, with carnitine and MCT oral supplementation. Treatment with riboflavin was not done because after delivery, she joined her family to Germany and was lost to follow-

Table 1 Clinical data, laboratory and genetic findings, and treatment

Patient no.	Gender	Age at onset (years)	Age at biopsy (years)	Causes of metabolic stress	Muscle carnitine levels (% of controls)	*ETFDH* gene mutations	Treatment
1	F	35	36	Poor nutrition and alcoholism	11	**c.412C>T, p.L138F,** exon 4; c.1531G>A, p. D511N, exon 12	Riboflavin (200 mg/day), carnitine (4 g/day), and carbamazepine
2	F	38	41	Poor nutrition	17	c.560C>T, p.A187V, exon 5; **c.1027T>C, p. W343R,** exon 11	Carnitine (2 g/day), MCT oil, riboflavin (200 mg/day), and steroids
3	F[a]	23	23	Hypoglycaemia, venous thrombosis, and weight loss	30	**c.451A>G (p. T151A),** exon 4 **c.1649T>G, p. L550P,** exon 12,	Heparin (5,000 U/L), 10% glucose i.v., riboflavin (200 mg/day), and carnitine (2 g/day)
4	F[a]	24	28	Sepsis and immunosuppressive treatment	12		Steroids, riboflavin, and methotrexate/cell-cept
5	F[b]	16	16	Pregnancy and delivery	10	c.152G>A (p.R51Q), exon 2	Carnitine (2 g/day) and steroids
6	M[b]	33	33	Cold exposure	20	**c.606+5insT,** exon 5	Riboflavin (200 mg/day)

Novel mutations are indicated in bold
[a,b] Pairs of siblings

up. We learned about her death from her brother, reporting that she was hospitalized for a respiratory infection, followed by a Reye-like syndrome. Steroid treatment was tried, but she went into coma and died at age 17 years.

Patient 6

This is the 33-year-old brother of patient 5. After being exposed to cold, he presented painful myalgia in the calves that progressed in the following days and extended to the thigh muscles. He could only walk 100 m because his lower limbs were swollen and stiff. CK was 3670 U/L and a first muscle biopsy showed LSM. Mitochondrial enzymes activities were reduced, after normalization to citrate synthase: NADH-dehydrogenase = 226.8 (normal values 391–663 nmol/min non-collagen protein), Succinate-dehydrogenase = 2.1 (n.v. 6.5–20.9), and Cytochrome oxidase = 14.71 (n.v. 24.5–57.5). A second muscle biopsy was performed, and mitochondria were isolated to conduct beta-oxidation studies, which showed a low oxidation of radiolabelled palmitate. Mitochondrial enzyme activities returned to be in the range of controls. On exercise tests with VO_{2max}, he arrived only to 60 W. He was then started

on riboflavin treatment at 200 mg/day, which resulted in a remarkable clinical improvement. A few months later, a second exercise test was normal.

Results

Patients

The clinical features of patients are summarized in Table 1. All patients had a juvenile/adult onset form with generalized muscle weakness, low muscle carnitine, and lipid storage in muscle, mostly localized in type 1 fibres. A variable decrease of OX-PHOS complexes documented mitochondrial involvement. Muscle ultrastructural analysis showed a massive increase of intra-cytoplasmic lipid droplets, which were usually localized nearby mitochondria and were found decreased after treatment.

Muscle Imaging

Muscle mass was investigated by imaging in three cases. By CT scan, an asymmetric atrophy of the legs was found

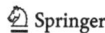

in patient 2, whereas by muscle MRI, there was atrophy of both in upper and lower girdle muscles and in leg muscles in patient 3, and irregular muscle mass and some fatty replacement in patient 4 (Fig. 1).

Genetic Analysis

Eight different mutations in the *ETFDH* gene have been identified (Table 1): four missense mutations are novel (p. L138F, p.T151A, p.W343R, and p.L550P), and three missense (p.R51Q [rs534388496], p.A187V [rs369912835], and p.D511N) have already been reported (Wen et al. 2010, 2013; Sugai et al. 2012). Moreover, a new splice site mutation has been detected in patient 6 (c.606+5insT). It is likely that his sister (patient 5), with a similar clinical and pathological features, might have carried the same mutations. Novel mutations have been confirmed by restriction enzyme analysis and not found in about 100 control chromosomes.

Discussion

Most patients with MADD have a good response to carnitine and riboflavin (Wen et al. 2010). Olsen et al. (2007) noted that riboflavin-responsive MADD may result from a defect in ETFDH, which might be associated with a generalized mitochondrial dysfunction. In support to this notion, all our patients had mutations in the *ETFDH* gene, and variable decrease of OX-PHOS complexes.

Table 2 summarizes the clinical differences between the different defects of FAs metabolism, as a guideline for subsequent studies. In RR-MADD, there is a characteristic profile of acyl-carnitines in blood (Wen et al. 2010) and concomitant low free carnitine in plasma and muscle.

Using the information from our cases, we developed a possible flow chart to make a diagnosis, since when secondary carnitine deficiency is suspected, L-carnitine supplementation brings a normal carnitine profile. Genetic analysis is important for the final diagnosis, since riboflavin can be added. Indeed, if clinical manifestations respond, it is worth undertaking ETFDH analysis, a common cause of MADD (Olsen et al. 2007).

It is noteworthy that an increased autophagic activity was found in our patients' muscle biopsies, which we previously found by immunoblot experiments (Angelini et al. 2016). In two of our patients, we previously demonstrated a co-localized expression of TFEB and p62/SQSTM1 (marker of protein aggregates) in atrophic fibres. Immunoblot analysis of p62/SQSTM1, LC3, and TFEB showed a marked increased expression during the acute phase of the disease. The appearance of a lipidated LC3-II band implies the occurrence of autophagosome prolifera-

Table 2 Clinical guidelines for screening defects of fatty acid metabolism

	Phenotype			
Enzyme/cofactor	Myopathy, hypotonia	Cardiomyopathy	Myoglobinuria	Hypoglycaemia, hypoketonaemia
Fatty acid transport				
Carnitine (*OCTN2* gene mutations)	++	++	−	++
Carnitine palmitoyl transferase	±	+	++	+
Beta-oxidation enzymes				
Long-chain acyl-CoA dehydrogenase	++	+	+	++
Medium-chain acyl-CoA dehydrogenase	±	±	−	++
Short-chain acyl-CoA dehydrogenase	+	±	−	+
3-Hydroxy acyl-CoA dehydrogenase	+	++	−	++
Neutral lipid storage (NLS) diseases				
NLSD-M	++	+	−	−
NLSD-I	+	−	−	−
Transferring flavoproteins				
Electron transfer flavoprotein (ETF)	±	±	−	++
ETF coenzyme Q reductase (ETF-QO)	±	−	−	++
Riboflavin-responsive forms (RR-MADD)	+	−	−	++

++ present, + sometimes present, ± rarely observed, − absent

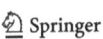

tion, while the concurrent increased p62/SQSTM1 expression was suggestive of a block of the autophagic flux (Angelini et al. 2016).

Other conditions such as neutral LSM (NLSD, due to *PNPLA2* or *ABDH5* gene mutations) do not recover, due to their lipolysis block. Unsurprisingly, NLSD patients present a variety of clinical manifestations, such as myopathy, hepatomegaly, and neuropathy, and respond poorly to treatment (Missaglia et al. 2015).

The data presented suggest that disturbances of mitochondrial protein integrity are a secondary consequence of RR-MADD. It is possible that the primary ETFDH deficiency may cause secondary impairment of mitochondrial OX-PHOS complexes due to accumulation of toxic metabolites and increased oxidative stress. Cornelius et al. (2012) observed a prolonged association of mutant ETFDH proteins in fibroblasts from such patients with the Hsp60 chaperon in mitochondrial matrix determining decreased heat stability. Risk factors to be considered in such patients are feverish state, bacterial or viral infections, physiological stresses like pregnancy, and restricted diet. Mitochondrial OX-PHOS status in macrophages during such metabolic crises is turned to an activated state resulting in a different metabolic anaerobic profile and increased ROS production (Angelini 2017; Mills et al. 2016).

An acute metabolic decompensation was fatal in patient 5, who had low muscle and plasma levels of carnitine, and LSM presumably for decreased oxidation of FAs and died of sepsis. Her brother presented a similar syndrome, but we were able to detect early his LSM with a low oxidation of radiolabelled palmitate in muscle and were able to treat his catabolic state.

A subgroup of patients with MADD showed a significant response to supplementary treatment with riboflavin, resulting in near-normalized biochemical and clinical parameters after high doses of oral supplementation: they are commonly referred as riboflavin-responsive MADD. This clinical entity has probably various aetiologies, that can be clinically differentiated from the primary SCD since patients present weakness of upper and lower girdle muscles, but no cardiomyopathy. The cause of the acute myopathy seems to be due to activation of lipophagy and block of metabolism, and lack of coenzyme FAD might result in instability of dehydrogenases, as observed in fibroblast cultures (Indo et al. 1991; Freneaux et al. 1992; Cornelius et al. 2012).

Synopsis

Here, six new cases of LSM with various phenotypes and precipitating factors are presented, with mutations of the *ETFDH* gene.

Conflict of Interest

Corrado Angelini declares that he has no conflict of interest. Daniela Tavian declares that she has no conflict of interest. Sara Missaglia declares that she has no conflict of interest.

Informed Consent

Informed consent was obtained from all patients for being included in the study.

Animal Rights

This article does not contain any studies with animals performed by any of the Authors.

Details of the Contribution of Individual Authors

Dr. Angelini collected and analysed the data, planned the study and wrote the manuscript. Drs. Tavian and Missaglia collected and analysed the data, and revised the manuscript.

References

Angelini C (2017) Metabolites-mitochondria-macrophages (MMM): new therapeutic avenues for inflammation and muscle atrophy. Transl Cancer Res 5(4):S8–S11 doi: 10.21037/tcr.2017.01.37

Angelini C, Govoni E, Bragaglia MM, Vergani L (1978) Carnitine deficiency: acute postpartum crisis. Ann Neurol 4:558–561

Angelini C, Nascimbeni AC, Cenacchi G, Tasca E (2016) Lipolysis and lipophagy in lipid storage myopathies. Biochim Biophys Acta 1862:1367–1373

Cornelius N, Frerman FE, Corydon TJ et al (2012) Molecular mechanism of riboflavin-responsiveness in patients with ETF-QO variations and multiple acyl-CoA dehydrogenation deficiency. Hum Mol Genet 21:3435–3448

Freneaux E, Sheffield VC, Molin L, Shires A, Rhead WJ (1992) Glutaric acidemia type II: heterogeneity in beta-oxidation flux, polypeptide synthesis, and complementary DNA mutations in the alpha-subunit of electron transfer flavoprotein in eight patients. J Clin Invest 90:1679–1686

Indo Y, Glassberg R, Yokota I, Tanaka K (1991) Molecular characterization of variant alpha-subunit of electron transfer flavoprotein in three patients with glutaric acidemia type II and identification of glycine substitution for valine 157 in the sequence of the precursor, producing an unstable mature protein in a patient. Am J Hum Genet 49:575–580

Liang WC, Nishino I (2011) Lipid storage myopathy. Curr Neurol Neurosci Rep 11:97–103

Mills EL, Kelly B, Logan A et al (2016) Succinate dehydrogenase supports metabolic repurposing of mitochondria to drive inflammatory macrophages. Cell 167:457–470

Missaglia S, Tasca E, Angelini C, Moro L, Tavian D (2015) Novel missense mutations in PNPLA2 causing late onset and clinical heterogeneity of neutral lipid storage disease with myopathy in three siblings. Mol Genet Metab 115:110–117

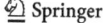

Olsen RK, Olpin SE, Andersen BS et al (2007) ETFDH mutations as a major cause of riboflavin-responsive multiple acyl-CoA dehydrogenase deficiency. Brain 130:2045–2054

Sugai F, Baba K, Toyooka K et al (2012) Adult-onset multiple acyl CoA dehydrogenation deficiency associated with an abnormal isoenzyme pattern of serum lactate dehydrogenase. Neuromuscul Disord 22:159–161

Wen B, Dai T, Li W et al (2010) Riboflavin-responsive lipid storage myopathy caused by ETFDH gene mutations. J Neurol Neurosurg Psychiatry 81:231–236

Wen B, Li D, Shan J et al (2013) Increased muscle coenzyme Q10 in riboflavin responsive MADD with ETFDH gene mutations due to secondary mitochondrial proliferation. Mol Genet Metab 109:154–160

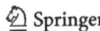

JIMD Reports
DOI 10.1007/8904_2017_24

RESEARCH REPORT

Successful Management of Pregnancies in Patients with Inherited Disorders of Ketone Body Metabolism

Raashda Ainuddin Sulaiman · Maha Al-Nemer ·
Rubina Khan · Munirah Almasned ·
Bedour S. Handoum · Zuhair N. Al-Hassnan

Received: 06 March 2017 / Revised: 27 March 2017 / Accepted: 28 March 2017 / Published online: 10 May 2017
© SSIEM and Springer-Verlag Berlin Heidelberg 2017

Abstract Patients with succinyl-CoA:3-oxoacid CoA transferase (SCOT) deficiency and 3-hydroxy-3-methylglutaryl (HMG)-CoA lyase deficiency are at increased risk of developing metabolic acidosis and hypoglycemia during pregnancy, delivery, and postpartum period. This can be fatal if not treated appropriately. Pregnancy in such patients should be managed in a specialist center by a multidisciplinary team including metabolic physician, high-risk obstetrician, and metabolic dietician. We report two pregnancies in women with SCOT deficiency and HMG-CoA lyase deficiency, which were successfully managed at this tertiary care center. The patient with SCOT deficiency had recurrent ketoacidosis due to severe nausea and vomiting requiring several hospital admissions during pregnancy, while the patient with HMG-CoA lyase deficiency remained metabolically stable. Both patients, nevertheless, had normal delivery of live-born infants and had uneventful postpartum period.

Communicated by: Avihu Boneh, MD, PhD, FRACP

R. A. Sulaiman (✉) · Z. N. Al-Hassnan
Department of Medical Genetics, King Faisal Specialist Hospital and Research Centre, Riyadh, Saudi Arabia
e-mail: rsulaiman@kfshrc.edu.sa

R. A. Sulaiman · Z. N. Al-Hassnan
College of Medicine, Alfaisal University, Riyadh, Saudi Arabia

M. Al-Nemer · R. Khan
Department of Obstetrics and Gynecology, King Faisal Specialist Hospital and Research Centre, Riyadh, Saudi Arabia

M. Almasned · B. S. Handoum
Department of Nutrition Services, King Faisal Specialist Hospital and Research Centre, Riyadh, Saudi Arabia

Introduction

Ketone bodies – acetoacetate and 3-hydroxybutyrate are the main sources of energy to the brain during fasting. These are produced mainly in the liver mitochondria from fatty acids and certain amino acids such as leucine, by the enzymes 3-hydroxy-3-methylglutaryl (HMG)-coenzyme A synthase and 3-hydroxy-3-methylglutaryl (HMG)-coenzyme A lyase which also catalyzes leucine degradation. Ketone bodies are metabolized in the peripheral tissues into acetyl CoA which enters Krebs cycle for energy production. The rate-limiting enzyme for ketolysis is succinyl-coenzyme A:3-oxoacid coenzyme A transferase (SCOT) (Fukao et al. 2014). HMG-CoA lyase deficiency (OMIM 613898) results in an inherited defect of ketogenesis and leucine degradation, while SCOT deficiency (OMIM 245050) causes an inherited defect of ketolysis. These patients develop acute metabolic crisis during fasting, febrile illness, infection, vomiting, diarrhea, or excessive physical exertion. During metabolic decompensation, patients with HMG-CoA lyase deficiency present with hypoketotic hypoglycemia, metabolic acidosis, and hyperammonemia, while those with SCOT deficiency present with severe ketoacidosis (Fukao et al. 2014). HMG-CoA lyase deficiency is relatively common in Saudi Arabia with an incidence of 1:55,357 in screened newborns (Ozand et al. 1991; Alfadhel et al. 2017). This is attributable to high consanguinity rate and the tribal structure in this population.

Early diagnosis and appropriate treatment of these disorders usually result in good long-term outcome with many patients reaching adulthood and pursuing goals of adult life. Pregnancy in these patients, however, carries a clear risk as nausea, vomiting, reduced oral intake, or excessive exertion may predispose them to severe, life-threatening crisis with metabolic acidosis and hypoglycemia. There are very limited data in the literature on the

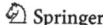

experience of managing these patients during pregnancy (Merron and Akhtar 2009; Langendonk et al. 2012; Pipitone et al. 2016). We report two successful pregnancies in women with SCOT deficiency and HMG-CoA lyase deficiency. We will discuss their management and the outcome of these pregnancies.

Case 1

A 19-year-old female with SCOT deficiency had recurrent episodes of ketoacidosis since the age of 2 years. The diagnosis was confirmed by molecular testing which revealed a previously reported homozygous mutation in *OXCT1* (c.1402C>T; p.R468C). She was on a protein-restricted, low-fat diet and L-carnitine supplements. The patient presented with severe nausea and vomiting at 6 weeks of gestation. She had ketoacidosis with serum bicarbonate level of 16 mmol/L. She was treated with intravenous 10% dextrose infusion in 0.45% saline with bicarbonate and potassium added in the infusion as required. Carnitine was initially given as intravenous injection (100 mg/kg body weight/day) as she could not tolerate medication or food orally. Her serum electrolytes and ammonia concentrations were monitored closely. She required ondansetron and later meclizine and metoclopramide for frequent vomiting. An ultrasound examination showed single viable fetus corresponding to dates. Maternal echocardiogram was unremarkable. She gradually improved over the next 3 weeks and started tolerating small, frequent, carbohydrate-rich, low-fat, mildly protein-restricted meals. She also had high-energy nutritional supplements (1–1.5 kcal/mL) orally as 100 mL every 3 h to provide 50–75% of her energy requirements. The patient was allowed 0.9 g/kg protein, with 15–23% fat in the diet, and was advised to use glucose polymers frequently during sick days and post vomiting. Since she lived in another town, a comprehensive antenatal care plan of her management including care during metabolic crisis and in labor as well as in the postpartum period was sent to her local physician. She had repeated admissions to the local hospital during rest of the pregnancy with excessive vomiting and ketoacidosis.

As her pregnancy advanced, the amount of daily protein intake was gradually increased to 1.3 g/kg daily with 30% calories from fat. She took carnitine as 100 mg/kg/day. Her complete blood count, renal profile, quantitative amino acids, prealbumin, zinc, selenium, and copper were monitored every month. She initially lost 4 kg in weight during the first trimester of pregnancy and then gradually gained 10 kg by 38 weeks of gestation. At 36 weeks gestation, an ultrasound examination for growth showed estimated fetal weight of 1.9 kg which was below fifth percentile for gestational age and confirmed intrauterine fetal growth restriction. She had elective induction of labor at 38.3 weeks gestation and delivered a female infant by normal vaginal delivery in our hospital. The baby's weight was 2.31 kg which was below third percentile for gestational age. During labor and delivery, she was given epidural anesthesia to avoid physiological stress of pain and received 10% dextrose in 0.45% saline with 20 mmol of bicarbonate in each liter of infusion, given at the rate of 80 mL/h. Carnitine was administered by intravenous injection as 100 mg/kg/day divided into 8 hourly doses. Serum electrolytes were monitored every 6 hourly during labor and then 12 hourly for next 48 h. Dextrose infusion with added sodium bicarbonate was continued for 24 h after delivery. She remained metabolically stable and breastfed her baby. She was discharged home three days after delivery.

Case 2

A 20-year-old female with HMG-CoA lyase deficiency was diagnosed at the age of 10 months when she presented with hypoglycemia and metabolic acidosis following gastroenteritis. She had homozygous mutation in *HMGCL* (c.122G>A; p.R41Q), a common pathogenic variant seen in Saudi patients. She was on a leucine-restricted diet, I-Valex-II (leucine-free protein supplement) and L-carnitine. She was a university student. There was no history of metabolic decompensation in the adult life. Although she had received prepregnancy counseling, she did not inform us about her pregnancy and attended an antenatal clinic at her local hospital. During her routine follow-up appointment in the metabolic clinic, she disclosed that she was 7 months pregnant. She had so far remained metabolically stable with uneventful pregnancy. Her blood test results showed hemoglobin of 94 g/L, serum bicarbonate 22 mmol/L, random blood glucose 4.4 mmol/L, and prealbumin level 140 mg/L (200–400). Plasma quantitative amino acid profile was unremarkable. The dose of carnitine was adjusted as 85 mg/kg/day. She continued on a leucine-restricted diet and restarted I-Valex-II which she had not been taking for the last 3 months since she ran out of stock. Her total protein intake was increased to 1.1 g/kg daily. She was advised to take glucose polymer (CarboCH) 96 g daily to meet her energy requirements. This patient was followed up in the high-risk pregnancy clinic for the remainder of her pregnancy. A month later, blood prealbumin levels improved to 250 mg/L, with normal amino acid levels, and hemoglobin was 104 g/L. She remained metabolically stable and gained

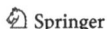

the desired 12.9 kg in weight by 38 weeks of pregnancy (prepregnancy BMI 16.2 kg/m^2). Her detailed care plan of management during pregnancy, labor, and postpartum period was made available in her electronic hospital records for easy access by the multidisciplinary team. She was electively induced at 38 week and 3 days of gestation. During labor she received 10% dextrose in 0.45% saline infusion with 20 mmol of sodium bicarbonate added to each liter and intravenous carnitine injections as in Case 1. She also received elective epidural anesthesia during labor. She delivered a healthy male infant by normal vaginal delivery. The baby's weight was 2.76 kg, at tenth percentile for the gestational age. The patient's blood electrolytes, ammonia, and glucose levels were monitored closely during labor and in the postpartum period as in Case 1. She remained well and was discharged home on the third day of delivery.

Discussion

These cases highlight the potential risks involved with pregnancies in women with inherited disorders of ketone body metabolism such as SCOT deficiency and HMG-CoA lyase deficiency. Nausea and vomiting of pregnancy cause problems in maintaining adequate caloric intake and compliance to medication. This may lead to severe metabolic decompensation in these patients, which, if not treated adequately, could lead to maternal and fetal loss (Langendonk et al. 2012). Such patients require prepregnancy counseling and preferably should have planned pregnancy, managed at the specialist center.

To date, there is only one published case report of pregnancy in a patient with SCOT deficiency who required hospitalization twice during pregnancy; however, labor and postpartum period were uneventful (Merron and Akhtar 2009). Pregnant women are known to have relative insulin resistance and demonstrate much higher blood levels of free fatty acids and β-hydroxybutyrate after fasting compared with nonpregnant women (Metzger et al. 1982). Starvation may precipitate ketoacidosis in pregnant women (Frise et al. 2013). Pregnant patients with SCOT deficiency are, therefore, at much higher risk of developing severe ketoacidosis even with mild nausea which restricts caloric intake. Ketone bodies readily cross the placenta and may harm the fetus in the presence of acidosis and dehydration. Our patient with SCOT deficiency had a history of frequent episodes of ketoacidosis during childhood and adolescence. She subsequently had a stormy course throughout her pregnancy with excessive nausea and vomiting culminating in several admissions to her local hospital with severe ketoacidosis. The patient was successfully managed during

these episodes in collaboration with her local physician. She, however, remained metabolically stable during the peripartum period.

The second case, a patient with HMG-CoA lyase deficiency is the first case report of an essentially uneventful pregnancy in a woman with this disorder, who successfully delivered a healthy boy. She remained metabolically stable and had no complications during pregnancy, labor, or postpartum. In the previously reported four pregnancies in two women with HMG-CoA lyase deficiency (Langendonk et al. 2012), there were two intrauterine fetal deaths, one termination of gestation and one maternal death. Although nausea and vomiting have been reported earlier as a specific problem in pregnancies with this particular disorder, our patient had minimal nausea and vomiting in early pregnancy which she tolerated very well without developing metabolic crisis.

Our patient with SCOT deficiency could not take adequate amount of calories and proteins due to intractable nausea and vomiting during most of her pregnancy. This, in addition to recurrent metabolic decompensations, led to the intrauterine fetal growth restriction. By contrast, fetal growth was not compromised in the patient with HMG-CoA lyase deficiency who managed to take her daily protein allowance and caloric requirement. Metabolic dieticians had regular telephonic contact with these patients and their nutritional requirements were constantly reviewed and modified with advancing pregnancy. The dose of carnitine was also adjusted as the pregnancy advanced. Both patients were followed up in the high-risk pregnancy clinic by obstetricians, in close collaboration with metabolic physicians and metabolic dieticians. They had elective induction of labor at around 38 weeks of gestation. Blood glucose, electrolytes, and ammonia levels were monitored closely during labor and after delivery. Prolonged high-dose oxytocin infusion was avoided as it may cause dilutional hyponatremia due to its antidiuretic effect. Pipitone et al. recently reported pregnancy in a patient with HMG-CoA lyase deficiency who developed metabolic acidosis due to overexertion during delivery (Pipitone et al. 2016). Our patients received elective epidural anesthesia in labor which saved them from physical stress and any related complication.

In summary management of these patients during pregnancy and delivery includes adequate caloric and protein intake with maintenance of hydration, electrolyte balance, and minimizing physiological stress of labor by giving epidural analgesia. The successful outcome in these two cases also reflects the importance of good collaboration in the multidisciplinary team, with a specific care plan in place preferably in the electronic patient record, to carefully

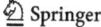
 Springer

monitor and manage these patients during pregnancy, labor, and postpartum for a successful outcome.

Acknowledgments We are thankful to Eman Megdad, Dana AlQasaby, and all the physicians for their contribution in the management of these patients.

Synopsis

Successful management of pregnancy and delivery in these patients includes multidisciplinary approach with maintenance of adequate caloric and protein intake, hydration, electrolyte balance, and minimizing physiological stress.

Details of the Contributions of Individual Authors

RAS, MN, and ZNH devised the prenatal and perinatal management protocol.

RAS participated in the management of both patients, planned, and wrote the manuscript.

ZNH, MN, RK, BSH, and MA participated in the management of patients and contributed to the manuscript.
Corresponding Author: Raashda A. Sulaiman.
Guarantor: Zuhair N. Al-Hassnan.

RAS, MN, RK, BSH, MA, and ZNH declare that they do not have any competing interest.

No funding was required for this report.

Informed consent has been taken from the patients.

References

Alfadhel M, Al Othaim A, Al Saif S et al (2017) Expanded newborn screening program in Saudi Arabia: incidence of screened disorders. J Paediatr Child Health. doi:10.1111/jpc.13469

Frise CJ, Mackillop L, Joash K et al (2013) Starvation ketoacidosis in pregnancy. Eur J Obstet Gynecol Reprod Biol 167(1):1–7

Fukao T, Mitchell G, Sass JO et al (2014) Ketone body metabolism and its defects. J Inherit Metab Dis 37:541–551

Langendonk JG, Roos JCP, Angus L et al (2012) A series of pregnancies in women with inherited metabolic disease. J Inherit Metab Dis 35:419–424

Merron S, Akhtar R (2009) Management and communication problems in a patient with succinyl-CoA transferase deficiency in pregnancy and labour. Int J Obstet Anesth 18(3):280–283

Metzger BE, Ravnikar V, Vileisis RA et al (1982) "Accelerated starvation" and the skipped breakfast in late normal pregnancy. Lancet 1:588–592

Ozand PT, Al Aqeel A, Gascon G et al (1991) 3-Hydroxy-3-methylglutaryl-coenzyme A (HMG-CoA) lyase deficiency in Saudi Arabia. J Inherit Metab Dis 14(2):174–188

Pipitone A, Raval DB, Duis J et al (2016) The management of pregnancy and delivery in 3-hydroxy-3-methylglutaryl-CoA lyase deficiency. Am J Med Genet A 170(6):1600–1602

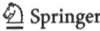

JIMD Reports
DOI 10.1007/8904_2017_28

Improvement of Fabry Disease-Related Gastrointestinal Symptoms in a Significant Proportion of Female Patients Treated with Agalsidase Beta: Data from the Fabry Registry

William R. Wilcox · Ulla Feldt-Rasmussen ·
Ana Maria Martins · Alberto Ortiz ·
Roberta M. Lemay · Ana Jovanovic ·
Dominique P. Germain · Carmen Varas ·
Katherine Nicholls · Frank Weidemann ·
Robert J. Hopkin

Received: 22 July 2016 / Revised: 11 April 2017 / Accepted: 18 April 2017 / Published online: 17 May 2017
© SSIEM and Springer-Verlag Berlin Heidelberg 2017

Abstract Fabry disease, an X-linked inherited lysosomal storage disorder, is caused by mutations in the gene encoding α-galactosidase, *GLA*. In patients with Fabry disease, glycosphingolipids accumulate in various cell types, triggering a range of cellular and tissue responses that result in a wide spectrum of organ involvement. Although variable, gastrointestinal symptoms are among the most common and significant early clinical manifestations; they tend to persist into adulthood if left untreated.

Communicated by: Ashok Vellodi

Electronic supplementary material: The online version of this chapter (doi:10.1007/8904_2017_28) contains supplementary material, which is available to authorized users.

W. R. Wilcox (✉)
Department of Human Genetics, Emory University School of Medicine, 615 Michael Street, Room 305H, Atlanta, GA 30322, USA
e-mail: william.wilcox@emory.edu

U. Feldt-Rasmussen
Department of Medical Endocrinology, Rigshospitalet, Copenhagen University Hospital, Copenhagen, Denmark

A. M. Martins
Reference Center for Inborn Errors of Metabolism, Federal University of São Paulo, São Paulo, Brazil

A. Ortiz
Unidad de Dialisis, IIS-Fundacion Jimenez Diaz, Universidad Autonoma de Madrid, Madrid, Spain

R. M. Lemay
Strategic Epidemiology and Biostatistics, Rare Diseases, Sanofi Genzyme, Cambridge, MA, USA

A. Jovanovic
Mark Holland Metabolic Unit, Salford Royal NHS Foundation Trust, Salford, UK

To further understand the effects of sustained enzyme replacement therapy (ERT) with agalsidase beta on gastrointestinal symptoms in heterozygotes, a data analysis of female patients enrolled in the Fabry Registry was conducted. To be included, females of any age must have received agalsidase beta (average dose 1.0 mg/kg every 2 weeks) for at least 2.5 years. Measured outcomes were self-reported gastrointestinal symptoms (abdominal pain, diarrhea). Outcomes at baseline and last follow-up, and their change from baseline to last follow-up, were assessed. Relevant data were available for 168 female patients. Mean age at the start of ERT was 43 years and mean treatment duration 5.7 years. Baseline pre-treatment abdominal pain was reported by 45% of females and diarrhea by 39%. At last follow-up, 31% reported abdominal pain ($p < 0.01$)

D. P. Germain
Division of Medical Genetics, University of Versailles – St Quentin en Yvelines, Paris-Saclay University, Montigny, France

C. Varas
Fabry Disease Multidisciplinary Team, Departamento Dermatología y ETS, Hospital San Pablo de Coquimbo, Coquimbo, Chile

K. Nicholls
Department of Nephrology, Royal Melbourne Hospital, Parkville, VIC, Australia

University of Melbourne, Parkville, VIC, Australia

F. Weidemann
Department of Internal Medicine II, Katharinen-Hospital Unna, Unna, Germany

R. J. Hopkin
Division of Human Genetics, Cincinnati Children's Hospital Medical Center, Cincinnati, OH, USA

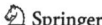

and 27% diarrhea ($p < 0.01$). The results of this Fabry Registry analysis suggest that while on sustained treatment with agalsidase beta (1.0 mg/kg every 2 weeks), both abdominal pain and diarrhea improved in many female patients with Fabry disease.

Introduction

Fabry disease (OMIM 301500) is an X-linked inherited lysosomal storage [123456]disorder caused by mutations in the *GLA* gene encoding the enzyme α-galactosidase (α-Gal) that lead to deficient or absent activity. This lack of activity results in the accumulation of globotriaosylceramide (GL-3) and other glycosphingolipids in the plasma and a variety of cell types including capillary endothelial, renal, cardiac, and nerve cells (Germain 2010). Glycolipid accumulation starts very early in life, is progressive, and triggers a range of cellular and tissue responses causing progressive damage to multiple organs. Life-threatening complications involving the kidneys, heart, and cerebrovascular system may start developing in the third decade of life (Wilcox et al. 2008; Germain 2010). The clinical presentation in female patients ranges from asymptomatic to, occasionally, a severe classic phenotype and depends in part on the mutation and the X-chromosome inactivation (Lyonization) profile (Germain 2010; Echevarria et al. 2016).

Gastrointestinal symptoms are among the most common and significant early clinical manifestations of Fabry disease, and may include abdominal pain, bloating, early satiety, intermittent/chronic diarrhea, constipation, recurrent nausea and vomiting, and poor weight gain (Ries et al. 2005; Ramaswami et al. 2006; Hoffmann et al. 2007; Hopkin et al. 2008; Buda et al. 2013; Politei et al. 2016). Studies among pediatric patients report abdominal pain as the most common gastrointestinal symptom (boys: 27–44%; girls: 17–27%) followed by diarrhea (boys: 19–33%; girls: 19–28%) (Ries et al. 2005; Ramaswami et al. 2006; Hopkin et al. 2008). Onset generally occurs earlier in boys than in girls (Ramaswami et al. 2006; Hopkin et al. 2008). These gastrointestinal symptoms tend to persist into adulthood if patients remain untreated (MacDermot et al. 2001; Hoffmann et al. 2007) and should therefore be assessed thoroughly and managed adequately to reduce their impact on quality of life.

Enzyme replacement therapies (ERTs) available for the treatment of patients with Fabry disease include agalsidase beta (Fabrazyme® [Sanofi Genzyme, Cambridge, MA, USA]; 1.0 mg/kg intravenously every 2 weeks) (Eng et al. 2001) and agalsidase alfa (Replagal® [Shire Human Genetic Therapies, Inc., Cambridge, MA, USA]; 0.2 mg/kg intrave-nously every 2 weeks) (Schiffmann et al. 2001). Both ERTs are available in the European Union and other countries worldwide, but only agalsidase beta is licensed in the USA.

To further understand the effects of sustained treatment with agalsidase beta treatment on gastrointestinal symptoms in female patients with Fabry disease, we analyzed data from the Fabry Registry.

Methods

The Fabry Registry (NCT00196742; sponsor: Sanofi Genzyme) is a multicenter, international, longitudinal, observational program designed to track the natural history and outcome of patients with Fabry disease (Eng et al. 2007; https://www.fabrycommunity.com/en/Healthcare/Registry.aspx). Patient and investigator participation is voluntary. To be included in the present Fabry Registry analysis, females of any age must have received agalsidase beta as their initial source of ERT given at the licensed dose of 1.0 mg/kg every 2 weeks (averaged dose; dose range: ≥0.9 to <1.1 mg/kg every 2 weeks), and have had a baseline (defined as time of first agalsidase beta infusion) and at least one additional on-treatment (i.e., follow-up after ≥2.5 years of agalsidase beta treatment) assessment of abdominal pain and/or diarrhea. The observation interval extended from the time each patient began treatment until one of the following occurred: (1) their most recently reported data to the Fabry Registry through April 3, 2015; (2) agalsidase beta treatment was discontinued; or (3) agalsidase beta treatment was switched to another treat-ment.

Data analyzed included age at first Fabry symptom, at diagnosis, and at first agalsidase beta infusion, and duration of agalsidase beta follow-up. Measured outcomes were self-reported gastrointestinal symptoms (abdominal pain, diar-rhea) since the last clinical assessment using responses "yes" [present] or "no" [not present] to the questions "Has the patient had abdominal pain since the last clinical assessment?" and "Has the patient had diarrhea since the last clinical assessment?" Patients were grouped by age at first agalsidase beta infusion: <30 years, 30–49 years, ≥50 years, and all ages; descriptive statistics were used to characterize the individuals within these age groups. Patients responding "yes" [present] or "no" [not present] at baseline and at ≥2.5 years of treatment were compared and p values calculated using a Chi-square distribution and the McNemar test statistic. Analyses of possible risk factors for lack of ERT response and occurrence of new gastroin-testinal symptoms included occurrence of severe clinical events (as defined elsewhere [Hopkin et al. 2016]) before or within the first 6 months of ERT, presence of estimated glomerular filtration rate (eGFR) values ≤60 mL/min/

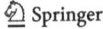

1.73 m^2 before or within the first 3 months of ERT (both chi-square), time from first symptom to first ERT, and time on ERT (both ANOVA). A p value <0.05 was considered to represent statistical significance. Statistical analyses were performed using SAS statistical software V.9.2 (SAS Institute, Cary, NC, USA).

Results

As of April 3, 2015 (cutoff date for the analysis), 2,564 female patients with Fabry disease had been enrolled in the Fabry Registry, of whom 895 had received agalsidase beta treatment and 168 had the data of interest (assessment of abdominal pain and/or diarrhea) at baseline and at ≥2.5 years of agalsidase beta treatment. Patient characteristics are summarized in Table 1. Of the 168 patients, 56% ($n = 94$) had a *GLA* mutation classified as "classic" in the Fabry disease mutation database (http://fabry-database.org/mutants/old.cgi) and 6% ($n = 10$) as later-onset mutations (p.N215S, $n = 5$; p.G35R; p.A97V; p.R112H; p.R301Q; p.I317T). Other mutations were either reported in the mutation database but not classified (10% [$n = 17$]) or not reported in the mutation database (14% [$n = 23$]). *GLA* mutations were not available for 14% ($n = 24$) of the patients.

Baseline and treatment follow-up data for abdominal pain and diarrhea are shown in Figs. 1 and 2, respectively. Significantly fewer patients reported abdominal pain at last follow-up than at baseline (45% vs. 31%, $p < 0.01$). Likewise, significantly fewer patients reported diarrhea at last follow-up compared with baseline (39% vs. 27%, $p < 0.01$). Of patients reporting abdominal pain or diarrhea at baseline, 55% and 57%, respectively, reported its absence at last follow-up. Of those reporting having no abdominal pain or diarrhea at baseline, 20% and 16%, respectively, reported its presence at last follow-up.

The effect of age and severity on ERT response and occurrence of new gastrointestinal symptoms was analyzed and is presented in Supplementary Tables S1 and S2.

Discussion

This analysis represents the longest longitudinal follow-up of the effect of ERT on gastrointestinal symptoms in the largest cohort of female patients with Fabry disease ($n = 168$) reported to date. In this Fabry Registry cohort, 45% of the females had reported abdominal pain and 39% diarrhea at the start of agalsidase beta treatment, with improvements to 31% and 27%, respectively, after a mean duration of ERT with agalsidase beta of 5.7 years. As our study included only patients initiated on treatment following baseline assessments, these incidences cannot be directly compared with data from studies on the natural history of Fabry disease. Moreover, percentages of gastrointestinal symptoms in female Fabry patients vary throughout the literature (MacDermot et al. 2001; Hoffmann et al. 2007;

Table 1 Baseline characteristics and ERT follow-up time for the 168 female Fabry patients who had abdominal pain (A) and/or diarrhea (B) status data available

(A) Abdominal pain

Age category for ERT initiation	Abdominal pain data available[a]	Age at first FD symptom, mean (SD)[b]	Age at FD diagnosis, mean (SD)[b]	Age at first ERT, mean (SD)	ERT follow-up time, mean (SD)
<30 years	32	11.5 (6.5)	16.3 (7.5)	20.8 (6.1)	5.4 (1.9)
30–49 years	75	17 (11.8)	34.1 (10.5)	41.1 (5.3)	5.7 (2.1)
≥50 years	59	31.7 (19.9)	50.9 (13.2)	58.2 (5.6)	5.8 (2.3)
Overall	166	20 (15.8)	36.5 (16.7)	43.3 (14.5)	5.7 (2.1)

(B) Diarrhea

Age category for ERT initiation	Diarrhea data available[a]	Age at first FD symptom, mean (SD)[b]	Age at FD diagnosis, mean (SD)[b]	Age at first ERT, mean (SD)	ERT follow-up time, mean (SD)
<30 years	32	11.5 (6.5)	16.3 (7.5)	20.8 (6.1)	5.5 (1.8)
30–49 years	71	17.5 (11.9)	34.6 (9.7)	41.1 (5.3)	5.8 (2.2)
≥50 years	57	31.2 (19.9)	50.5 (13.3)	58.2 (5.6)	5.8 (2.2)
Overall	160	19.9 (15.6)	36.5 (16.5)	43.1 (14.6)	5.7 (2.1)

ERT enzyme replacement therapy with agalsidase beta, *FD* Fabry disease, *SD* standard deviation
[a] Data available at baseline and ≥2.5 years of ERT
[b] Age at first Fabry disease symptom and age at Fabry disease diagnosis were not known for all included patients

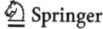

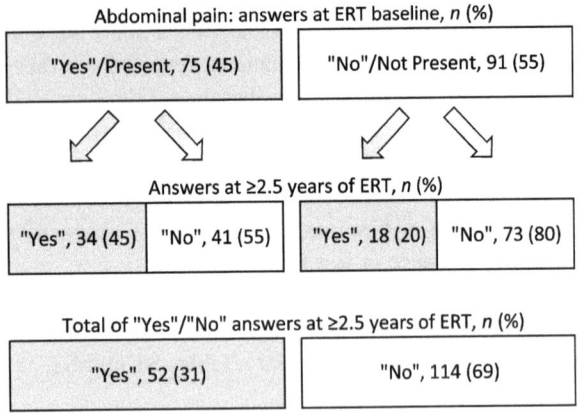

Fig. 1 Abdominal pain responses ("yes" [present] or "no" [not present]) from 166 females with Fabry disease at treatment baseline and at ≥2.5 years of ERT. *ERT* enzyme replacement therapy with agalsidase beta

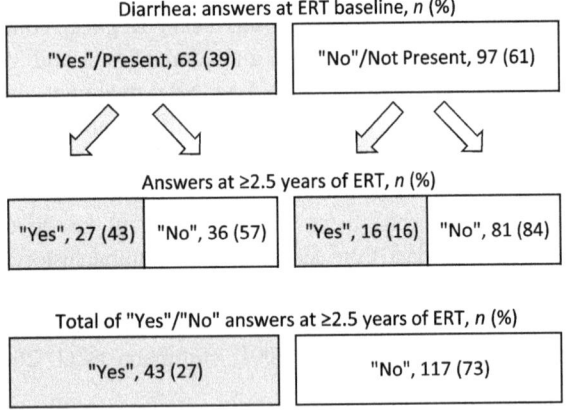

Fig. 2 Diarrhea responses ("yes" [present] or "no" [not present]) from 160 females with Fabry disease at treatment baseline and at ≥2.5 years of ERT. *ERT* enzyme replacement therapy with agalsidase beta

Pensabene et al. 2016). In comparison, although scarce, epidemiological data on different abdominal symptoms in normal populations suggest that gastrointestinal symptoms are common. One large Danish population study found 1-year incidences of abdominal pain to range from 43 to 55% among females aged 30–60 years, with the vast majority reporting having pain weekly, monthly, or less frequently (Kay et al. 1994).

Of the females reporting abdominal pain or diarrhea at baseline in our analysis, more than half did not report these symptoms at last follow-up. A minority of patients reported no gastrointestinal symptoms at baseline, but did report abdominal pain (20%) and diarrhea (16%) at last follow-up. Whether the new symptoms are due to Fabry disease or unrelated causes is unknown. In a supplemental analysis for the effects of age and disease severity on response to ERT, diarrhea was more persistent in women aged ≥50 years with eGFR values ≤60 mL/min/1.73 m^2 ($p < 0.01$,

Supplementary Table S2). Abdominal pain appeared during treatment more frequently in females aged 30–49 years who had been on ERT longer (5.1 vs. 6.8 years, $p = 0.04$, Supplementary Table S1). However, given the small sample size, the clinical significance of these findings remains unclear.

Several studies have reported improvements in gastrointestinal symptoms with ERT in both children and adult patients with Fabry disease (Banikazemi et al. 2005; Hoffmann et al. 2007; Wraith et al. 2008; Ramaswami et al. 2012). However, only one study reported ERT follow-up data for adult female patients separately (Hoffmann et al. 2007). This Fabry Outcome Survey registry study found that 2 years of agalsidase alfa treatment in 25 female patients reduced the incidence of abdominal pain from 40 to 20%, while the incidence of diarrhea increased compared with baseline (12–16%).

Knowledge about the pathophysiology of gastrointestinal symptoms in Fabry disease and mechanisms of action of ERT on these symptoms remains incomplete. Deposition of GL-3 in the mesenteric vascular endothelium, autonomic ganglia cells of Meissner's and Auerbach's plexus, and smooth muscle cells is believed to contribute to Fabry disease pathology in the gastrointestinal tract, and lead to endothelial dysfunction, vasculopathy, neuropathy, and myopathy, and subsequently to delayed gastric emptying and intestinal dysmotility (MacDermot et al. 2001; Buda et al. 2013).

Although data are lacking, it can be hypothesized that initiation of ERT exerts an effect on gastrointestinal symptoms by (partially) clearing GL-3 from cells in the gastrointestinal system and preserving cellular function or ameliorating cellular dysfunction. Complete clearance of GL-3 from endothelial cells and other cell types, improvement in small nerve fiber function, and quality of life have been reported in studies on agalsidase beta (Eng et al. 2001; Hilz et al. 2004; Germain et al. 2007; Watt et al. 2010). Indirect evidence suggests that a higher ERT dose may be of clinical benefit in ameliorating gastrointestinal symptoms. A recent study showed that patients treated with agalsidase alfa experienced more gastrointestinal pain than those treated with agalsidase beta (at reduced or licensed dose) (Lenders et al. 2016).

One of the challenges regarding the study of gastrointestinal symptoms in real-world clinical practice is that the symptoms evolve and change (e.g., progress and remit), making it difficult to design a study which would inarguably demonstrate that the response, or lack thereof, is due to the therapy rather than the passage of time or other factors. This holds especially for the study of female patients, where gastrointestinal symptoms before and during menses could be a confounder in studying these symptoms due to Fabry disease (Bernstein et al. 2014).

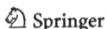

If gastrointestinal symptoms are the first and only manifestations, the diagnosis of Fabry disease may be challenging particularly if there is no positive family history. Misdiagnoses include irritable bowel syndrome, chronic inflammatory bowel disease (IBD), appendicitis, autoimmune disorders, Whipple's disease, dermatomyositis, Crohn's disease, celiac disease, and colon cancer (Buda et al. 2013; Politei et al. 2016). However, these medical conditions may coincide with Fabry disease, as Fabry patients in the authors' clinics have been correctly diagnosed with concomitant autoimmune IBD, lactose intolerance, gluten enteropathy, bacterial overgrowth, pancreatitis, neuroendocrine bowel tumor, and pheochromocytoma.

Limitations associated with using data from the Fabry Registry must be considered in the present analysis. Not all female patients with Fabry disease have been diagnosed and enrolled; however, it is likely that the more severely affected patients are being treated with ERT and are enrolled and followed in the Registry. The Fabry Registry contains observational data of Fabry patients only. It is not a prospective clinical trial and data interpretation is limited by the lack of an appropriately matched control group. For example, untreated women have not been analyzed to investigate how their gastrointestinal problems change over time. Relatively crude measures of self-reported abdominal pain and diarrhea have been used in the analysis, because sufficient data on change in frequency and intensity of abdominal pain and change in frequency of diarrhea are not available. These measures may be biased by recall, patient (mis)perception, and lack of specific definitions for the symptoms of interest. Although the Fabry Registry provides a recommended schedule of assessments, patients and treating physicians determine which assessments the patients will receive and the time intervals at which they will be conducted. Patients may have incompletely reported medical histories, may be lost to follow-up, or may have used concomitant medications to alleviate gastrointestinal symptoms. Finally, the analysis does not assess non-Fabry-related causes of gastrointestinal symptoms: sufficient data on the use of concomitant medications were not available for analysis, nor were patient records for other causes of gastrointestinal symptoms.

Conclusions

This analysis represents the longest longitudinal follow-up of the effect of ERT on gastrointestinal symptoms in the largest cohort of female patients with Fabry disease reported to date. Commonly reported gastrointestinal symptoms prior to initiation of agalsidase beta treatment included abdominal pain and diarrhea. The results of this Fabry Registry analysis suggest that sustained treatment with agalsidase beta (1.0 mg/kg every 2 weeks for a mean of 5.7 years) improves both abdominal pain and diarrhea in many female patients. Women who do not respond or who develop new abdominal symptoms on ERT should be investigated for alternate causes. Further studies are needed to better understand the pathology underlying the gastrointestinal symptoms and the mechanisms of action of ERT in the treatment of these symptoms. Gastrointestinal symptoms should be assessed thoroughly and managed adequately using available adjunctive therapies to reduce their impact on the patient's well-being.

Acknowledgments The authors would like to thank the many patients who have agreed to participate in the Fabry Registry as well as the physicians and research coordinators who have entered clinical data on behalf of these patients.

Synopsis

Enzyme replacement therapy with agalsidase beta alleviates both abdominal pain and diarrhea in a significant proportion of female patients with Fabry disease.

Compliance with Ethics Guidelines

Conflict of Interest

See the financial activities section below.

This research was funded by Sanofi Genzyme, the sponsor of the Fabry Registry.

Informed Consent

All procedures followed were in accordance with the ethical standards of the responsible committees on human experimentation (institutional and national) and with the Helsinki Declaration of 1975 (revised in 2000). Each independent Fabry Registry site is responsible for obtaining a patient's informed written consent to submit their health information to the Registry, and to use and disclose this information in subsequent aggregate analyses.

Author Contributions

William R. Wilcox, Ulla Feldt-Rasmussen, Alberto Ortiz, Dominique P. Germain, Frank Weidemann, and Robert J. Hopkin contributed to the concept/design of the manuscript, data acquisition, data analysis/interpretation, drafting the manuscript, and critically revising it.

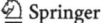

Ana Maria Martins, Ana Jovanovic, Carmen Varas, and Katherine Nicholls contributed to the data acquisition, data analysis/interpretation, drafting the manuscript, and critically revising it.

Roberta M. Lemay contributed to the concept/design of the manuscript, data analysis/interpretation, drafting the manuscript, and critically revising it.

Financial Relationships for the Work Under Consideration for Publication

The authors received medical writing/editing support in the preparation of this manuscript from Alessia Piazza and Tom Rouwette of Excerpta Medica, funded by Sanofi Genzyme. The authors also thank Hans Ebels for providing medical writing/editing services and Badari Gudivada for providing programming support on behalf of Sanofi Genzyme. A. Ortiz was supported by ISCIII intensificación de la actividad investigadora. This research was funded by Sanofi Genzyme, the sponsor of the Fabry Registry.

Relevant Financial Activities Outside the Submitted Work

- **William R. Wilcox** consults for Sanofi Genzyme and is an investigator in clinical studies and trials sponsored by Sanofi Genzyme, Shire HGT, Amicus Therapeutics, and Protalix Corporation. These activities are monitored and are in compliance with the conflict of interest policies at Emory University School of Medicine.
- **Ulla Feldt-Rasmussen** has received honoraria for lectures and participation in advisory boards from Sanofi Genzyme, Shire HGT, and Amicus Therapeutics, and has received research funds from Sanofi Genzyme and Shire HGT.
- **Ana Maria Martins** is a member of the Fabry Registry Board of Advisors and has received research funds, travel support, and speaking fees from Sanofi Genzyme.
- **Alberto Ortiz** is a consultant for Sanofi Genzyme and has received speaker fees from Shire HGT.
- **Roberta M. Lemay** is an employee of Sanofi Genzyme.
- **Ana Jovanovic** is a member of the Fabry Registry Board of Advisors and has received advisory board fees and honoraria for lectures from Sanofi Genzyme, Shire HGT, and Amicus Therapeutics.
- **Dominique P. Germain** is a consultant for Sanofi Genzyme and Shire HGT and has received honoraria for lectures from Sanofi Genzyme, Shire HGT, and Amicus Therapeutics.
- **Carmen Varas** is a member of the Fabry Registry Board of Advisors.
- **Katherine Nicholls** has received research support and travel grants from Sanofi Genzyme, Amicus Therapeutics, and Shire HGT, and speaker honoraria from Sanofi Genzyme and Shire HGT.
- **Frank Weidemann** has received speaker honoraria from Sanofi Genzyme and Shire HGT, is a member of the Fabry Registry European Board of Advisors, and has received travel assistance and speaker honoraria. Research grants were given to his institution by Sanofi Genzyme and Shire HGT.
- **Robert J. Hopkin** consults with Sanofi Genzyme and Shire HGT and has been an investigator in clinical trials sponsored by Sanofi Genzyme, Shire HGT, and Amicus Therapeutics. These activities have been monitored and found to be in compliance with the conflict of interest policies at Cincinnati Children's Hospital Medical Center.

References

Banikazemi M, Ullman T, Desnick RJ (2005) Gastrointestinal manifestations of Fabry disease: clinical response to enzyme replacement therapy. Mol Genet Metab 85:255–259

Bernstein MT, Graff LA, Avery L, Palatnick C, Parnerowski K, Targownik LE (2014) Gastrointestinal symptoms before and during menses in healthy women. BMC Womens Health 14:14

Buda P, Książyk J, Tylki-Szymanska A (2013) Gastroenterological complications of Anderson-Fabry disease. Curr Pharm Des 19:6009–6013

Echevarria L, Benistan K, Toussaint A et al (2016) X-chromosome inactivation in female patients with Fabry disease. Clin Genet 89:44–54

Eng CM, Fletcher J, Wilcox WR et al (2007) Fabry disease: baseline medical characteristics of a cohort of 1765 males and females in the Fabry Registry. J Inherit Metab Dis 30:184–192

Eng CM, Guffon N, Wilcox WR et al (2001) Safety and efficacy of recombinant human alpha-galactosidase A – replacement therapy in Fabry's disease. N Engl J Med 345:9–16

Fabry disease mutation database (H. Sakuraba). http://fabry-database.org/mutants/old.cgi. Accessed 7 Apr 2016

Germain DP (2010) Fabry disease. Orphanet J Rare Dis 5:30

Germain DP, Waldek S, Banikazemi M et al (2007) Sustained, long-term renal stabilization after 54 months of agalsidase beta therapy in patients with Fabry disease. J Am Soc Nephrol 18:1547–1557

Hilz MJ, Brys M, Marthol H, Stemper B, Dütsch M (2004) Enzyme replacement therapy improves function of C-, Adelta-, and Abeta-nerve fibers in Fabry neuropathy. Neurology 62:1066–1072

Hoffmann B, Schwarz M, Mehta A, Keshav S (2007) Gastrointestinal symptoms in 342 patients with Fabry disease: prevalence and response to enzyme replacement therapy. Clin Gastroenterol Hepatol 5:1447–1453

Hopkin RJ, Bissler J, Banikazemi M et al (2008) Characterization of Fabry disease in 352 pediatric patients in the Fabry Registry. Pediatr Res 64:550–555

Hopkin RJ, Cabrera G, Charrow J et al (2016) Risk factors for severe clinical events in male and female patients with Fabry disease treated with agalsidase beta enzyme replacement therapy: data from the Fabry Registry. Mol Genet Metab 119:151–159

Kay L, Jørgensen T, Jensen KH (1994) Epidemiology of abdominal symptoms in a random population: prevalence, incidence, and natural history. Eur J Epidemiol 10:559–566

Lenders M, Canaan-Kühl S, Krämer J et al (2016) Patients with Fabry disease after enzyme replacement therapy dose reduction and switch-2-year follow-up. J Am Soc Nephrol 27:952–962

MacDermot KD, Holmes A, Miners AH (2001) Anderson-Fabry disease: clinical manifestations and impact of disease in a cohort of 60 obligate carrier females. J Med Genet 38:769–775

Pensabene L, Sestito S, Nicoletti A, Graziano F, Strisciuglio P, Concolino D (2016) Gastrointestinal symptoms of patients with Fabry disease. Gastroenterol Res Pract 2016:9712831

Politei J, Thurberg BL, Wallace E, Warnock D, Serebrinsky G, Durand C, Schenone AB (2016) Gastrointestinal involvement in Fabry disease. So important, yet often neglected. Clin Genet 89:5–9

Ramaswami U, Whybra C, Parini R et al (2006) Clinical manifestations of Fabry disease in children: data from the Fabry Outcome Survey. Acta Paediatr 95:86–92

Ramaswami U, Parini R, Pintos-Morell G, Kalkum G, Kampmann C, Beck M (2012) Fabry disease in children and response to enzyme replacement therapy: results from the Fabry Outcome Survey. Clin Genet 81:485–490

Ries M, Gupta S, Moore DF et al (2005) Pediatric Fabry disease. Pediatrics 115:e344–e355

Schiffmann R, Kopp JB, Austin HA 3rd et al (2001) Enzyme replacement therapy in Fabry disease: a randomized controlled trial. JAMA 285:2743–2749

Watt T, Burlina AP, Cazzorla C et al (2010) Agalsidase beta treatment is associated with improved quality of life in patients with Fabry disease: findings from the Fabry Registry. Genet Med 12:703–712

Wilcox WR, Oliveira JP, Hopkin RJ et al (2008) Females with Fabry disease frequently have major organ involvement: lessons from the Fabry Registry. Mol Genet Metab 93:112–128

Wraith JE, Tylki-Szymanska A, Guffon N et al (2008) Safety and efficacy of enzyme replacement therapy with agalsidase beta: an international, open-label study in pediatric patients with Fabry disease. J Pediatr 152:563–570

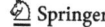

JIMD Reports
DOI 10.1007/8904_2017_30

RESEARCH REPORT

Ketone Bodies as a Possible Adjuvant to Ketogenic Diet in PDHc Deficiency but Not in GLUT1 Deficiency

F. Habarou · N. Bahi-Buisson · E. Lebigot ·
C. Pontoizeau · M. T. Abi-Warde · A. Brassier ·
K. H. Le Quan Sang · C. Broissand ·
S. Vuillaumier-Barrot · A. Roubertie · A. Boutron ·
C. Ottolenghi · P. de Lonlay

Received: 08 March 2017 / Revised: 23 April 2017 / Accepted: 26 April 2017 / Published online: 17 May 2017
© SSIEM and Springer-Verlag Berlin Heidelberg 2017

Abstract *Objective*: Ketogenic diet is the first line therapy for neurological symptoms associated with pyruvate dehydrogenase deficiency (PDHD) and intractable seizures in a number of disorders, including GLUT1 deficiency syndrome (GLUT1-DS). Because high-fat diet raises serious compliance issues, we investigated if oral L,D-3-hydroxybutyrate administration could be as effective as ketogenic diet in PDHD and GLUT1-DS.

Methods: We designed a partial or total progressive substitution of KD with L,D-3-hydroxybutyrate in three GLUT1-DS and two PDHD patients.

Results: In GLUT1-DS patients, we observed clinical deterioration including increased frequency of seizures and myoclonus. In parallel, ketone bodies in CSF decreased after introducing 3-hydroxybutyrate. By contrast, two patients with PDHD showed clinical improvement as dystonic crises and fatigability decreased under basal metabolic conditions. In one of the two PDHD children, 3-hydroxybutyrate has largely replaced the ketogenic diet, with the latter that is mostly resumed only during febrile illness. Positive direct effects on energy metabolism in PDHD patients were suggested by negative correlation between ketonemia and lactatemia ($r^2 = 0.59$). Moreover, in cultured PDHc-deficient fibroblasts, the increase of CO_2 production after ^{14}C-labeled 3-hydroxybutyrate supplementation was consistent with improved Krebs cycle activity. However, except in one patient, ketonemia tended to be lower with 3-hydroxybutyrate administration compared to ketogenic diet.

Conclusion: 3-hydroxybutyrate may be an adjuvant treatment to ketogenic diet in PDHD but not in GLUT1-DS under basal metabolic conditions. Nevertheless, ketogenic diet is still necessary in PDHD patients during febrile illness.

Communicated by: Uma Ramaswami

F. Habarou · C. Pontoizeau · C. Ottolenghi
Metabolic Biochemistry Department, Necker Enfants Malades Hospital, AP-HP, Paris Descartes University, Inserm U1124, Paris, France

N. Bahi-Buisson
Department of Neurology, Necker Enfants Malades Hospital, AP-HP, Imagine Institute, Paris Descartes University, Paris, France

E. Lebigot · A. Boutron
Department of Biochemistry, Bicêtre Hospital, AP-HP, Paris, France

M. T. Abi-Warde
Department of Neuropediatrics, Strasbourg Hospital, Strasbourg, France

A. Brassier · P. de Lonlay (✉)
Reference Center of Inherited Metabolic Diseases, Necker Enfants Malades Hospital, AP-HP, Imagine Institute, University Paris Descartes, Paris, France
e-mail: pascale.delonlay@aphp.fr

K. H. Le Quan Sang
Department of Genetics, Necker Enfants Malades Hospital, AP-HP, Imagine Institute, Paris Descartes University, Paris, France

C. Broissand
Department of Pharmacy, Necker Enfants Malades Hospital, AP-HP, Paris, France

S. Vuillaumier-Barrot
Department of Biochemistry, Bichat Hospital, AP-HP, Paris, France

A. Roubertie
Department of Neuropediatrics, Gui de Chauliac Hospital, INSERM U-1051, Institute for Neuroscience of Montpellier, Montpellier, France

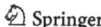

Introduction

Pyruvate dehydrogenase complex deficiency (PDHD) and GLUT1 deficiency syndrome (GLUT1-DS) are two energetic diseases, respectively caused by a deficiency of any component of the PDHc (E1α (OMIM 312170), E1β (OMIM 614111), E2 (OMIM 245348), E3 (OMIM 246900) or E3BP (OMIM 245349)), or heterozygous mutations/deletions in *SLC2A1* gene (OMIM 606777). Both diseases lead to impairment of glucose metabolism, an essential energetic substrate, by defect in either pyruvate oxidation in mitochondria or glucose transport across the blood–brain barrier (BBB) and astrocytes. Patients have neurological involvement, ranging from severe encephalopathy to later and milder symptoms such as dystonia (Patel et al. 2012; Hully et al. 2015; De Giorgis et al. 2016).

Because ketone bodies (KB), a source of acetyl-CoA, can compensate for energetic defect in PDHD and GLUT-1DS, ketogenic diet (KD), a high-fat, low-carbohydrate and normal protein diet is the first line treatment for both diseases, with a global improvement in neurological condition in PDHD (Barnerias et al. 2010). Seizure control is obtained within a week to a month in most GLUT1-DS patients (Klepper et al. 2005) while improvement in other paroxysmal symptoms is poorly documented (Leen et al. 2010).

A major limit of KD is its unpallability and side effects (digestive symptoms, nephrolithiasis, hyperlipidemia, osteopenia) (Klein et al. 2014). Indeed, the classical KD contains from 70% (1/1KD) to 90% (4/1KD) of fat. Our aim was to substitute partially or totally KD with L,D-3-hydroxybutyrate in three GLUT1-DS patients and two PDHD patients in order to improve patients quality of life and compliance. The results were highly divergent, with an

improvement for PDHD patients in basal conditions, which contrasted with worsening of GLUT1-DS patients.

Patients and Methods

Patients

GLUT1-DS Patients

Hypoglycorrachia, decreased CSF/blood glucose ratio, and heterozygous mutation/deletion in the *SLC2A1* gene led to GLUT1-DS diagnosis in the three patients (P) (Table 1).

P1 presented with early onset epileptic encephalopathy. GLUT1-DS was diagnosed at age 2 years.

P2 presented early onset myoclonic epilepsy, spastic cerebellar syndrome, and psychomotor delay. Diagnosis was performed at age 11 years.

P3 presented with neonatal hypotonia, strabismus, and abnormal head movements. He worsened with fasting and had "absences" in the morning. At age 5 years, psychomotor delay, pharmacoresistant epilepsy, abnormal movements, and dystonia led to the diagnosis.

PDHD Patients

P4, a girl, started fever-induced episodes of fatigue at age 8 months. At age 3 years, right leg dystonic crises appeared, whose frequency increased progressively: they occurred daily, were exercise-induced, and involved the right half of the body and the left foot. Psychomotor development was normal. She developed a peripheral neuropathy. At age 7 years, cerebral MRI showed dentate nucleus and globi pallidi hypersignals and corpus callosum

Table 1 Genetic and biochemical findings in three GLUT1-DS and two PDHc-deficient patients

	Genetic findings	Biochemical findings
Patient 1 (current age 11 years)	De novo complete *SLC2A1* deletion	Glycorrachia: 1.9 mmol/L Glycemia: 4.2 mmol/L CSF/Blood glucose: 0.45
Patient 2 (current age 22 years)	*SLC2A1* Exon 4 c.436G>A p.Glu146Lys	Glycorrachia: 1.7 mmol/L Glycemia: 6.8 mmol/L CSF/Blood glucose: 0.25
Patient 3 (current age 12 years)	*SLC2A1* Exon 1 c.32_33delGC p.Arg11fProfs[a]77	Glycorrachia: 1.4 mmol/L Glycemia: 4.7 mmol/L CSF/Blood glucose: 0.3
Patient 4 (current age 15 years)	*PDHA1* Exon 8 c.787C>G p.Arg263Gly	PDH activity[a]: 2,069 pmol/min/mg of protein
Patient 5 (current age 12 years)	*PDHA1* Exon 7 c.650C>G p.Pro217Arg	PDH activity[a]: 785 pmol/min/mg of protein

[a] PDH activity was measured in lymphocytes. Normal range: 1,570–3,430 pmol/min/mg of proteins

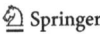

abnormalities suggesting the diagnosis of PDHD. A previously described mutation in *PDHA1* was identified (Table 1) (Imbard et al. 2011). PDHc activity measured in lymphocytes was within normal range (Table 1), due to the X-chromosome inactivation bias in tissues (Matthews et al. 1994).

P5, a boy, presented with peripheral neuropathy, cerebellar syndrome, and episodes of fatigability. A de novo mutation in *PDHA1* was found at age 3 years, and PDHc activity was decreased in lymphocytes (Table 1).

Methods

Treatments

Clinical presentation and initial treatments were variable among patients, whose number was limited. Patients were chosen for their symptoms easy to parameterize and because of parents' will to test an alternative to KD. L,D-3-hydroxybutyrate sodium salt (INRESA, Bartenheim, France) was mixed with water and given three times daily. Treatment's clinical effectiveness was evaluated by occurrence and frequency of seizures for P1, P2, and P3, and by dystonia crises or fatigability episodes frequency (pallor, very hypotonic, sleeping) for P4 and P5, respectively, thanks to notes taken daily by parents and educators.

Ketone Bodies, Lactate, and PDHc Activity Measurement

Blood/CSF KB concentrations and lactatemia were measured on a Konelab 30 analyzer (Vassault et al. 1991). Urinary 3-hydroxybutyrate was assayed by gas chromatography-mass spectrometry with standard clinical laboratory methods. PDHc activity was carried out as described (Imbard et al. 2011).

In Vitro Oxidation Rate Measurement

Oxidation rates of 3-hydroxybutyrate and glucose were measured after incubation with 10 mM 1-^{14}C labeled substrates in cultured fibroblasts from a control and an unrelated PDHD patient presenting with an intermittent strabismus and an axial hypotonia related to a de novo mutation in *PDHA1* (p.Arg378His) (Imbard et al. 2011). Fibroblasts from GLUT1-DS patients were not available.

Results

Clinical Follow-Up

In GLUT1-DS P1 to P3, treatments consisted first in 3/1 or 4/1KD alone then 4/1 to 2/1KD associated with increasing

doses of L,D 3-hydroxybutyrate (from 400 to 1,200 mg/kg/day). Under 3/1 or 4/1KD, the number of generalized seizures dramatically decreased. However, the partial substitution of KD with L,D-3-hydroxybutyrate led to clinical deterioration (Fig. 1).

In P1, at diagnosis, a 3/1 then 4/1KD was established and 250 mg/day valproic acid was introduced, which allowed to control seizures except in context of poor compliance. Under KD, only a motor improvement was noticed. Under 2/1KD and 800 mg/kg/day L,D-3-hydroxybutyrate, myoclonus/seizure reoccurred on a monthly basis. A 1/1KD and 1,200 mg/kg/day L,D-3-hydroxybutyrate combination led to equilibrium disorders and seizures crises. As a precursor of succinyl-CoA and as such an anaplerotic compound, valine supplementation was transiently attempted but was inefficient.

In P2, 4/1KD was started at age 12 years and controlled myoclonus. Combinations of 3/1KD and various doses of L,D-3-hydroxybutyrate led to increased myoclonus (up to once a day under 3/1KD and 1,080 mg/kg/day L,D-3-hydroxybutyrate) and seizure (up to 1–2 crises per month under 3/1KD and 700 mg/kg/day L,D-3-hydroxybutyrate) frequency. An acute worsening happened with the combination of 2/1KD and 900 mg/kg/day L,D-3-hydroxybutyrate, leading us to switch to 3/1KD and 900 mg/kg/day L,D-3-hydroxybutyrate. As precursors of succinyl-CoA and oxaloacetate, respectively, valine and aspartate were given but without effect.

In P3, absences disappeared under 3/1KD, soon established after diagnosis. After 1-day interruption in KD, he experienced increased fatigability without any abnormal movement, whereas after several days movement disorders reoccurred. Of note, absences and seizures were still under control. Combinations of 3/1KD and from 500 to 1,140 mg/kg/day L,D-3-hydroxybutyrate were well-tolerated, without any change in his condition. When a 2/1KD with 900–1,200 mg/kg/day L,D-3-hydroxybutyrate was established, his condition worsened with the reappearance of seizures and 3–4 absences every morning.

All patients stopped L,D-3-hydroxybutyrate administration and were moved back to their initial KD treatment, respectively, 4/1KD for P1 and P2 and 3/1KD for P3. They recovered their initial condition.

The two PDHD patients showed a dramatically positive response. We designed either a total (in P4) or partial (in P5) substitution of KD with L,D-3-hydroxybutyrate. In basal conditions, this suppressed the dystonic crisis in P4, and strongly reduced fatigability in P5 (Fig. 2).

In P4, 1/1KD and 100 mg/day thiamine decreased the dystonic crises frequency from 3 per day to 1–2 per week depending on physical activities. A 1/1KD associated with 500 mg/kg/day L,D-3-hydroxybutyrate was well-tolerated and as efficient as 1/1KD alone. The increase of L,D-3-

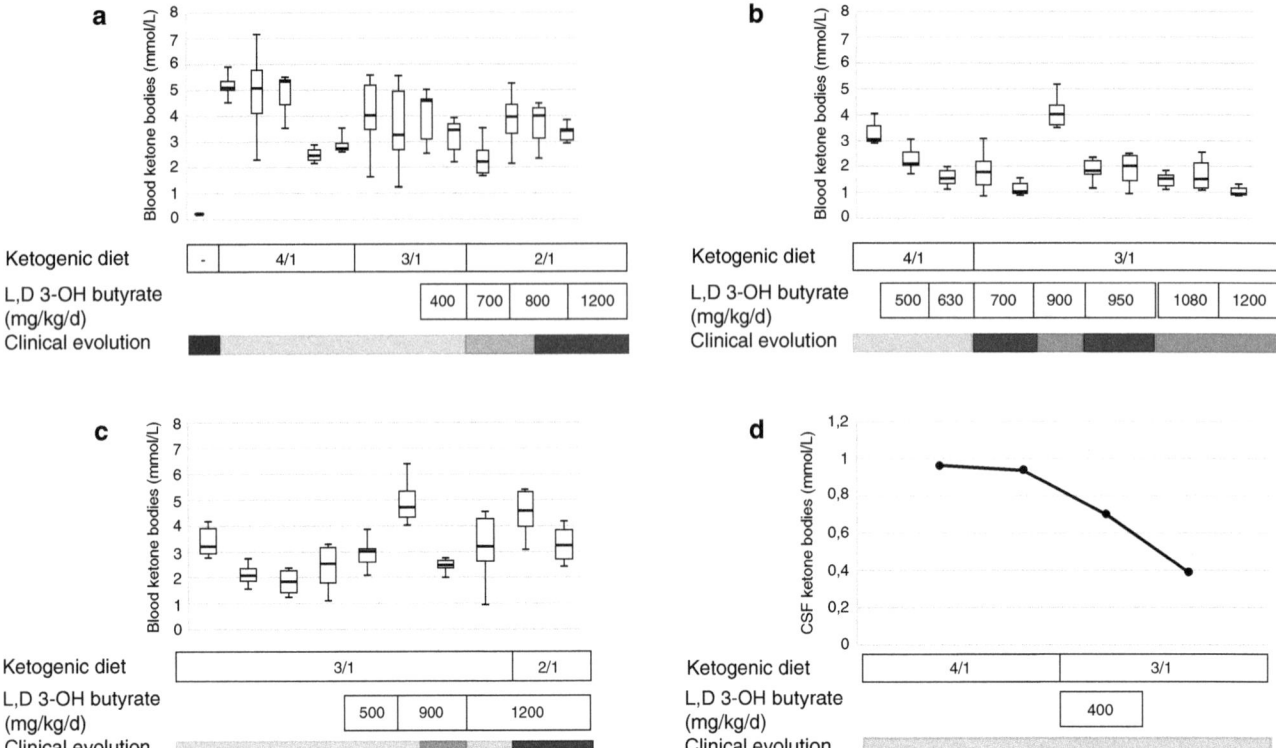

Fig. 1 Biological investigations, treatments, and clinical evolution in GLUT1-DS patients. (**a**, **b**, **c**) Ketonemia, treatments and clinical evolution in 3 GLUT1-DS patients (**a**: patient 1; **b**: patient 2; **c**: patient 3). *Boxplots* show median, minimum, maximum, first and third quartiles of ketonemia. (**d**) CSF ketone bodies and clinical evolution in patient 1. For each patient, the total duration of partial KD substitution with L,D-3-hydroxybutyrate was about 2 years. Clinical evolution was evaluated based on frequency of myoclonus or seizures. Clinical condition worsening was represented by *darker rectangles*

hydroxybutyrate up to 900 mg/kg/day improved her condition, with only one dystonic crisis a month. Then a "less than 1/1KD" was started with up to 1,200 mg/kg/day L,D-3-hydroxybutyrate: one to two dystonic crises occurred monthly, favored by walking. Finally, KD was stopped: 1,000–1,200 mg/kg/day L,D-3-hydroxybutyrate controlled dystonia crises under basal conditions.

Under 2/1 or 3/1KD during illness and 100 mg/day thiamine, P5 had several fatigability episodes per week. First, a combination of 3/1KD and 500 mg/kg/day L,D-3-hydroxybutyrate was established and well-tolerated during few days, with improved condition. Then a degradation event occurred outside any febrile episode: he was very tired, his legs were painful, he dribbled and could not drink, with an unchanged appetite. Finally he recovered soon. Under 2/1KD and 500 mg/kg/day L,D-3-hydroxybutyrate, fatigability episodes occurred daily, but were less intense than before. Then 1/1KD and doses of L,D-3-hydroxybutyrate ranging from 700 to 900 mg/kg/day improved his condition. No overt fatigability episodes were recorded. Recently, he developed episodes of right leg dystonia in a context of poor compliance. During fever, a 3/1 to 4/1KD was transiently administered whereas oral KB administration was ineffective on clinical symptoms.

Biological Follow-Up

In GLUT1-DS patients, the different treatments allowed to maintain a sustained ketosis. Mean ketonemia was 3.53 (Standard Deviation (SD): 1.49) in P1, 2.08 (SD: 1.03) in P2, and 3.17 (SD: 1.22) in P3 (Fig. 1a–c), all concentrations in mmol/L. However, the highest ketonemias were measured under 4/1KD. CSF ketone bodies concentrations, in mmol/L, ranged in P1 between 0.39 and 0.96 under 3/1 or 4/1KD alone, respectively, (mean: 0.76; SD: 0.32), and reached 0.7 under 3/1KD with 400 mg/kg/day L,D-3-hydroxybutyrate (Fig. 1d). The highest CSF ketone bodies concentration was measured under 4/1KD (Fig. 1d).

In PDHD patients, mean ketonemia, in mmol/L, was milder: 0.32 (SD: 0.22) in P4, and 1.82 (SD: 0.95) in patient 5 (Fig. 2a, b). Of note, lactatemia correlates negatively with ketonemia ($r^2 = 0.39$ in patient 4; $r^2 = 0.59$ in patient 5; Fig. 2c, d). Under L,D-3-hydroxybutyrate and KD association, ketonemias tended to be lower than under KD alone. Ketonuria was highly variable under the different treatments in GLUT1-DS and PDHD patients (data not shown). Mean blood free fatty acids levels were, in mmol/L, 0.82 (SD: 0.34) in GLUT1-DS patients, and 0.62 (SD: 0.47) in PDHD patients.

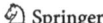

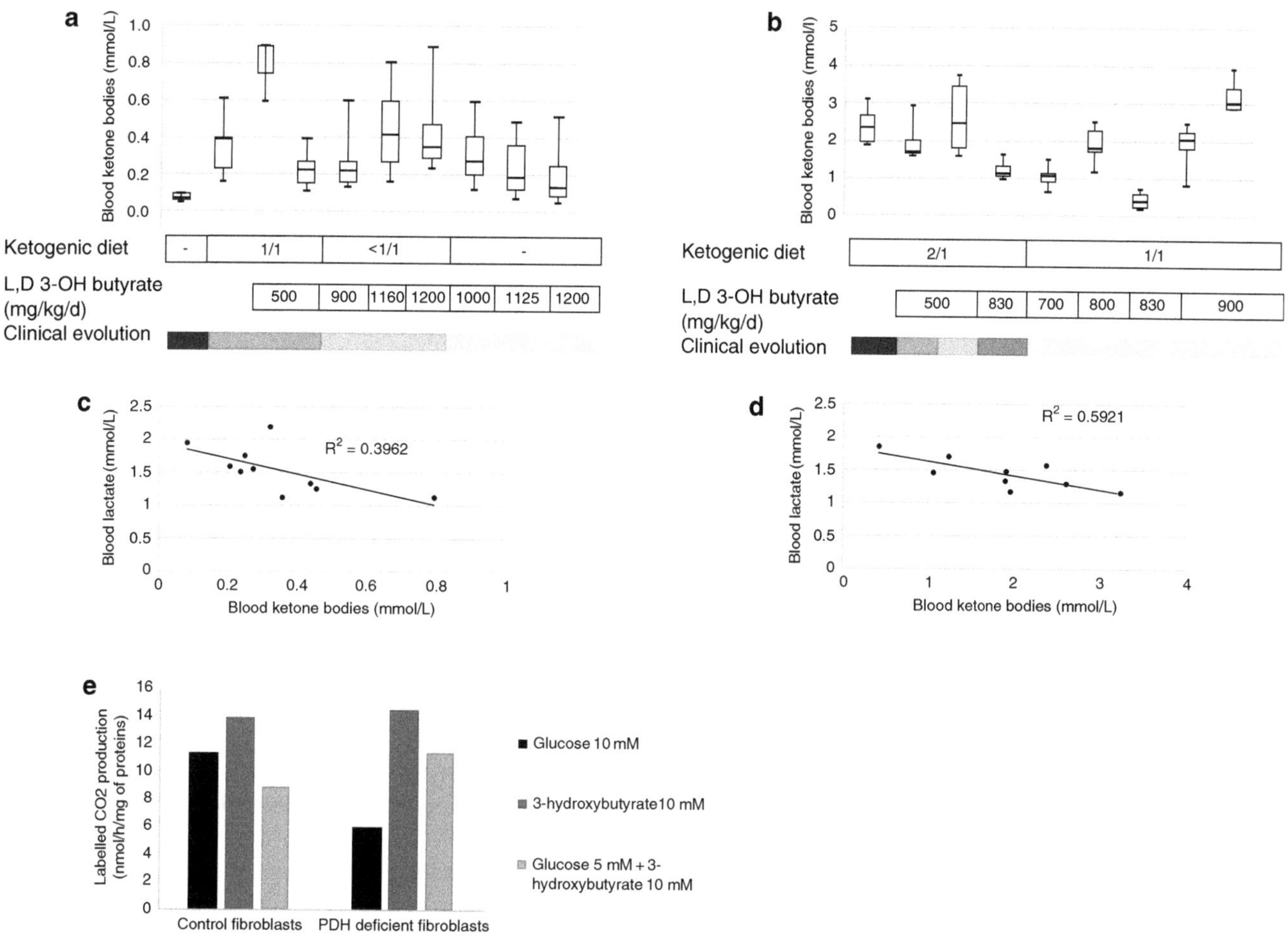

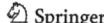

Fig. 2 Biological investigations, treatments, and clinical evolution in PDHc-deficient patients, and in vitro study of 3-hydroxybutyrate and glucose oxidation ability in PDHD fibroblasts. (**a**, **b**) Ketonemia, treatment and clinical evolution in two PDHc-deficient patients (**a**: patient 4; **b**: patient 5). *Boxplots* show median, minimum, maximum, first and third quartiles of ketonemia. Clinical evolution was evaluated based on frequency of dystonic crises or fatigability. Clinical condition worsening was represented by *darker rectangles*. (**c**, **d**) Correlation between lactatemia and ketonemia in two PDHc-deficient patients (**c**: patient 4; **d**: patient 5). (**e**) CO_2 production in control and PDHc-deficient fibroblasts using glucose and/or 3-hydroxybutyrate as substrates

In Vitro Study of 3-Hydroxybutyrate and Glucose Oxidation Ability in PDHD Fibroblasts

In PDHD fibroblasts, CO_2 production from glucose was decreased by half, consistent with impaired glucose oxidation (Fig. 2e). PDHD cells were able to oxidize 3-hydroxybutyrate as efficiently as in control, either alone or in combination with glucose, consistent with increased Krebs cycle activity because of PDHc-independent production of acetyl-CoA from 3-hydroxybutyrate.

Discussion

This study was designed as a proof of concept test for any added value of KB in PDHD and GLUT1-DS treatment. To improve quality of life and compliance, we tried to replace KD partially or totally with L,D-3-hydroxybutyrate in three GLUT1-DS and two PDHD patients. The clinical evolution of GLUT1-DS and PDHD patients was strikingly different. In all GLUT1-DS patients, a partial replacement of KD with L,D-3-hydroxybutyrate led to clinical degradation. Conversely, a positive effect of KB administration was obvious in two PDHD patients although KD was still necessary when energetic needs increase, for example, during febrile illness periods.

Interestingly, in our GLUT1-DS patients, oral 3-hydroxybutyrate administration was unable to raise blood and CSF KB concentrations as high as 4/1 or 3/1KD (see Fig. 1c). CSF 3-hydroxybutyrate concentrations were comparable to those described by Klepper et al. in 5 GLUT1-DS under 3/1KD (Klepper et al. 2004).

According to Morris, the major determinants of brain KB metabolism are blood KB concentration and availability of suitable monocarboxylate transporters (MCT) (Morris 2005). However, in our patients, there was no obvious correlation between clinical condition and ketonemia, as previously reported (Freeman et al. 2006). Oral administration of KB might inhibit ketogenic synthesis (Balasse and Neef 1975). KB is produced in liver and exported into blood through MCT1 and 2, transported across the BBB via MCT1, and taken up by neurons and astrocytes via MCT1 or MCT2 (Halestrap and Wilson 2012). MCT1 and GLUT1 expression increased in brain of rats fed with high-fat diet for 6 weeks (Leino et al. 2001). MCT2 mRNA was reported to increase after a 48 h food deprivation (Matsuyama et al. 2009). Pan et al. highlighted the importance of 3-hydroxybutyrate transport induction: after 3-hydroxybutyrate infusion, brain 3-hydroxybutyrate concentrations were lower than those measured in fasted adults (Pan et al. 2001). By reducing KD, perhaps a less important induction of MCT1 and GLUT1 was achieved, leading to decreased energetic substrates availability in brain. Our three GLUT1-DS patients might have been more sensitive to such a regulatory process than our two PDHD patients.

Our findings illustrate the dual function of glucose as supplier of acetyl-CoA and Krebs cycle intermediates. Both these functions are presumably impaired in GLUT1-DS whereas only acetyl-CoA production is reduced in PDHD. Under KD, glycolysis and glucose oxidative metabolism decrease. In PDHD patients, when KD was less restrictive or suppressed, glycolysis might re-increase. Glucose-derived pyruvate may enter the Krebs cycle via pyruvate carboxylase (PC), thus ensuring 3-hydroxybutyrate-derived acetyl-CoA combustion. Of note, KD and 3-hydroxybutyrate have been shown to stimulate pyruvate carboxylation and thus Krebs cycle anaplerosis (Melo et al. 2006), as they supply cells with acetyl-CoA, a well-known activator of PC. In PDHD-patients, combination of a less restrictive KD with L,D-3-hydroxybutyrate might have led not only to increased "fuel" (acetyl-CoA) oxidation but also to increased anaplerosis through PC in astrocytes, a process probably impaired in GLUT1-DS due to glucose transport impairment across the BBB and astrocyte membrane.

This point might be particularly important since seizures are thought to cause a deficiency in Krebs cycle intermediates, especially oxalo-acetate and alpha-ketoglutarate (Melo et al. 2005). Our study suggests that an anaplerotic mechanism may be involved because in PDHD patients, lactatemia correlates negatively with ketonemia (Fig. 2).

If anaplerosis is indeed defective in GLUT1-DS, the use of triheptanoin, a heptanoate triglyceride which can provide acetyl-CoA and propionyl-CoA, might be interesting as recently described (Pascual et al. 2014; Mochel et al. 2016). Combinations of 3-hydroxybutyrate with other anaplerotic compounds (such as multiple amino acids) may also be considered.

In conclusion, the clinical condition improved in two PDHD patients when we attempted to replace KD with L,D-3-hydroxybutyrate, arguing for a direct beneficial effect of KB in this energetic disease. However, KD was still necessary during febrile illness episodes and more patients would be necessary to confirm our finding before any recommendation. By contrast, GLUT1-DS patients worsened with increased seizures or myoclonus frequency, suggesting that additional metabolic processes, possibly Krebs cycle anaplerosis and mechanisms unrelated to energy metabolism, may be affected.

Take-Home Message

3-Hydroxybutyrate may be used as an adjuvant to ketogenic diet in PDHD, not in GLUT1-DS, and only under basal metabolic conditions.

Contribution of Individual Authors

Acquisition, analysis, interpretation of data: *F. Habarou, E. Lebigot, A. Boutron, S. Vuillaumier-Barrot, C. Pontoizeau, C. Ottolenghi, P. de Lonlay.*

Clinical work and treatment supervision: *N. Bahi-Buisson, M.T. Abi-Warde, A. Brassier, A. Roubertie, K.H. Le Quan Sang, C. Broissand, P. de Lonlay.*

Drafting of the manuscript: *F. Habarou, C. Ottolenghi, P. de Lonlay.*

Critical revision of the manuscript: *all authors.*

Corresponding Author

Pr Pascale de Lonlay, Reference Center of Inherited Metabolic Diseases, Necker Enfants Malades Hospital, AP-HP, 149 rue de Sèvres, 75015 Paris, France; pascale. delonlay@aphp.fr.

Competing Interest Statement

F. Habarou, N. Bahi-Buisson, E. Lebigot, C. Pontoizeau, M.T. Abi-Warde, A. Brassier, K.H. Le Quan Sang, C. Broissand, S. Vuillaumier-Barrot, A. Roubertie, A. Boutron, C. Ottolenghi, and P. de Lonlay declare that they have no conflict of interest.

This work is academic. It was carried out by clinicians and biologists independent of any pharmaceutical company.

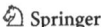

Funding

The authors did not receive any specific private financial support for the research, authorship, and/or publication of this article. We thank the "Jérôme Lejeune" foundation (2014), and Associations of Families (Nos Anges, AMMI, Noa Luu, Hyperinsulinisme).

Ethics Approval and Patient Consent

This work was approved by our institutional ethical committee after declaration to the *Département de la Recherche Clinique et du Développement*, and informed consent was obtained from the parents.

References

Balasse E, Neef M (1975) Inhibition of ketogenesis by ketone bodies in fasting humans. Metabolism 24:999–1007

Barnerias C, Saudubray J, Touati G, De Lonlay P, Dulac O, Ponsot G, Marsac C, Brivet M, Desguerre I (2010) Pyruvate dehydrogenase complex deficiency: four neurological phenotypes with different pathogenesis. Dev Med Child Neurol 52:e1–e9

De Giorgis V, Varesio C, Baldassari C, Piazza E, Olivotto S, Macasaet J, Balottin U, Veggiotti P (2016) Atypical manifestations in GLUT1 deficiency syndrome. J Child Neurol 31:1174–1180

Freeman J, Veggiotti P, Lanzi G, Tagliabue A, Perucca E (2006) The ketogenic diet: from molecular mechanisms to clinical effects. Epilepsy Res 68:145–180

Halestrap A, Wilson M (2012) The monocarboxylate transporter family–role and regulation. IUBMB Life 64:109–119

Hully M, Vuillaumier-Barrot S, Le Bizec C, Boddaert N, Kaminska A, Lascelles K, De Lonlay P, Cances C, des Portes V, Roubertie A, Doummar D, LeBihannic A, Degos B, de Saint Martin A, Flori E, Pedespan J, Goldenberg A, Vanhulle C, Bekri S, Roubergue A, Heron B, Cournelle M, Kuster A, Chenouard A, Loiseau M, Valayannopoulos V, Chemaly N, Gitiaux C, Seta N, Bahi-Buisson N (2015) From splitting GLUT1 deficiency syndrome to overlapping phenotypes. Eur J Med Genet 58:443–454

Imbard A, Boutron A, Vequaud C, Zater M, De Lonlay P, De Baulny H, Barnerias C, Miné M, Marsac C, Saudubray J, Brivet M (2011) Molecular characterization of 82 patients with pyruvate dehydrogenase complex deficiency. Structural implications of novel amino acid substitutions in E1 protein. Mol Genet Metab 104:507–516

Klein P, Tyrlikova I, Mathews G (2014) Dietary treatment in adults with refractory epilepsy. Neurology 83:1978–1985

Klepper J, Diefenbach S, Kohlschütter A, Voit T (2004) Effects of the ketogenic diet in the glucose transporter 1 deficiency syndrome. Prostaglandins Leukot Essent Fatty Acids 70:321–327

Klepper J, Scheffer H, Leiendecker B, Gertsen E, Binder S, Leferink M, Hertzberg C, Näke A, Voit T, Willemsen M (2005) Seizure control and acceptance of the ketogenic diet in GLUT1 deficiency syndrome: a 2- to 5-year follow-up of 15 children enrolled prospectively. Neuropediatrics 36:302–308

Leen W, Klepper J, Verbeek M, Leferink M, Hofste T, van Engelen B (2010) Glucose transporter-1 deficiency syndrome: the expanding clinical and genetic spectrum of a treatable disorder. Brain 133:655–670

Leino R, Gerhart D, Duelli R, Enerson B, Drewes L (2001) Diet-induced ketosis increases monocarboxylate transporter (MCT1) levels in rat brain. Neurochem Int 38:519–527

Matsuyama S, Ohkura S, Iwata K, Uenoyama Y, Tsukamura H, Maeda K, Kimura K (2009) Food deprivation induces monocarboxylate transporter 2 expression in the brainstem of female rat. J Reprod Dev 55:256–261

Matthews P, Brown R, Otero L, Marchington D, LeGris M, Howes R, Meadows L, Shevell M, Scriver C, Brown G (1994) PDH deficiency: clinical presentation and molecular genetic characterization of five new patients. Brain 117:435–443

Melo T, Nehlig A, Sonnewald U (2005) Metabolism is normal in astrocytes in chronically epileptic rats: a (13)C NMR study of neuronal-glial interactions in a model of temporal lobe epilepsy. J Cereb Blood Flow Metab 25:1254–1264

Melo T, Nehlig A, Sonnewald U (2006) Neuronal-glial interactions in rats fed a ketogenic diet. Neurochem Int 48:498–507

Mochel F, Hainque E, Gras D, Adanyeguh IM, Caillet S, Heron B, Roubertie A, Kaphan E, Valabregue R, Rinaldi D, Vuillaumier-Barrot S, Schiffmann R, Ottolenghi C, Hogrel J, Servais L, Roze E (2016) Triheptanoin dramatically reduces paroxysmal motor disorder in patients with GLUT1 deficiency. J Neurol Neurosurg Psychiatry 87:550–553

Morris A (2005) Cerebral ketone body metabolism. J Inherit Metab Dis 28:109–121

Pan J, Telang F, Lee J, de Graaf R, Rothman D, Stein D, Hetherington H (2001) Measurement of beta-hydroxybutyrate in acute hyper-ketonemia in human brain. J Neurochem 79:539–544

Pascual JM, Liu P, Mao D, Kelly DI, Hernandez A, Sheng M, Good L, Ma Q, Marin-Valencia I, Zhang Z, Park J, Hynan L, Stavinoha P, Roe C, Lu H (2014) Triheptanoin for glucose transporter type I deficiency (G1D): modulation of human ictogenesis, cerebral metabolic rate, and cognitive indices by a food supplement. JAMA Neurol 71:1255–1265

Patel K, O'Brien T, Subramony S, Shuster J, Stacpoole P (2012) The spectrum of pyruvate dehydrogenase complex deficiency: clinical, biochemical and genetic features in 371 patients. Mol Genet Metab 106:385–394

Vassault A, Bonnefont J, Specola N, Saudubray J (1991) Lactate, pyruvate, and ketone bodies. In: Homme FA (ed) Techniques in diagnostic human biochemical genetics: a laboratory manual. Wiley Liss, New York, pp 285–308

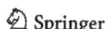

JIMD Reports
DOI 10.1007/8904_2017_31

RESEARCH REPORT

GM2 Activator Deficiency Caused by a Homozygous Exon 2 Deletion in *GM2A*

Patricia L. Hall · Regina Laine · John J. Alexander ·
Arunkanth Ankala · Lisa A. Teot · Hart G. W. Lidov ·
Irina Anselm

Received: 27 November 2016 / Revised: 19 March 2017 / Accepted: 2 May 2017 / Published online: 25 May 2017
© SSIEM and Springer-Verlag Berlin Heidelberg 2017

Abstract GM2 activator (GM2A) deficiency (OMIM 613109) is a rare lysosomal storage disorder, with onset typically in infancy or early childhood. Clinically, it is almost indistinguishable from Tay-Sachs disease (OMIM 272800) or Sandhoff disease (OMIM 268800); however, traditionally available biochemical screening tests will most likely reveal normal results. We report a 2-year-old male with initially normal development until the age of 9 months, when he presented with developmental delay and regression. Workup at that time was unrevealing; at 15 months, he had abnormal brain MRI findings and a cherry red spot on ophthalmological examination. Family history and all laboratory studies were uninformative. The combination of a cherry red spot and developmental regression was strongly suggestive of a lysosomal storage disorder. Sequence analysis of *GM2A* did not reveal any pathogenic variants; however, exon 2 of *GM2A* could not be amplified by PCR, raising suspicion for a large, homozygous deletion. Subsequent copy number analysis confirmed a homozygous deletion of exon 2 in *GM2A*. This is the first reported case of GM2A deficiency being caused by a whole exon deletion. We describe previously unreported electron microscopy findings in this disease, thus expanding the clinical and variant spectrum for GM2 activator deficiency. These findings demonstrate the increased degree of suspicion required for diagnosis of this rare disorder.

Brief Summary: This case of GM2 activator deficiency was caused by a homozygous deletion in *GM2A*, demonstrating the need to include exon level copy number analysis in any workup to fully exclude this disorder.

Communicated by: Marc Patterson

Patricia L. Hall and Regina Laine contributed equally to this work.

P. L. Hall (✉) · J. J. Alexander · A. Ankala
Department of Human Genetics, Emory University, Atlanta, GA 30322, USA
e-mail: patricia.l.hall@emory.edu

P. L. Hall · J. J. Alexander · A. Ankala
EGL Genetics, Tucker, GA 30084, USA

R. Laine
Department of Neurology, Mitochondrial Program, Neuromuscular Program, Boston Children's Hospital, Boston, MA 02115, USA

L. A. Teot
Department of Pathology, Boston Children's Hospital, Boston, MA 02115, USA

H. G. W. Lidov
Department of Pathology, Neuropathology, Boston Children's Hospital, Boston, MA 02115, USA

H. G. W. Lidov
Pathology, Harvard Medical School, Boston, MA 02115, USA

I. Anselm
Department of Neurology, Mitochondrial Program, Boston Children's Hospital, Boston, MA 02115, USA

I. Anselm
Neurology, Harvard Medical School, Boston, MA 02115, USA

Introduction

Complete degradation of gangliosides in human cells requires proper function of three gene products: *HEXA*, *HEXB*, and *GM2A*. Pathogenic variants in *HEXA* and *HEXB* cause Tay-Sachs and Sandhoff disease, respectively, conditions which can be easily identified by a variety of biochemical assays, including enzyme analysis for both and urine oligosaccharide screening for Sandhoff disease (Xia et al. 2013; Hall et al. 2014). Tay-Sachs disease and Sandhoff disease are caused by defective subunits of the hexosamini-

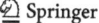

dase enzyme. Variants in *GM2A* cause a clinical phenotype indistinguishable from infantile Tay-Sachs or Sandhoff disease; however, there is no readily available biochemical assay for the identification of this condition. Identification and diagnosis requires a high degree of suspicion and persistence, despite consistently normal or uninformative results. At present, only a small number of patients have been reported and all of these are of infantile onset (Schroder et al. 1993; Schepers et al. 1996; Sakuraba et al. 1999; Smith et al. 2012; Renaud and Brodsky 2015). A 2015 summary of available literature identified fewer than ten published cases of molecularly confirmed GM2A deficiency (Renaud and Brodsky 2015).

Case Report

A 2-year-old male was evaluated in our clinic for loss of milestones and a cherry red spot on ophthalmological exam. Pregnancy and delivery were uncomplicated. Both parents are Chinese, with no known consanguinity. Earliest milestones were achieved at a normal time including rolling over and sitting. The first concerns were around 8 or 9 months of age, when the child was not advancing and had lost the ability to babble and reach for toys. At the time, the workup included EMG, EEG, and pelvic CT, all of which were unremarkable. Initial MRI at 15 months of age showed abnormal T2 hyper-intensities in the basal ganglia and also periventricular white matter changes. An ophthalmology exam revealed a cherry red spot. At this time, a karyotype was performed which was normal and lysosomal enzyme assay results were all within normal limits. Family history was noncontributory for any similarly affected individuals. The patient underwent extensive genetic testing

in China, including a sequencing panel for metabolic disorders which included several disorders associated with the clinical finding of a cherry red spot, including Tay-Sachs disease and Sandhoff disease, but not GM2 activator deficiency.

At 2 years of age, he was unable to crawl or sit independently, and could no longer roll over. He was nondysmorphic, normocephalic without organomegaly, had excessive startle reflex, was irritable, non-verbal, made no eye contact, and did not track objects. He had axial hypotonia and profound weakness, brisk deep tendon reflexes, but no Babinski sign. The cherry red spot was confirmed at this time and repeat lysosomal enzyme testing was normal. Further metabolic workup including lactic acid, acylcarnitine, amino acids, urine organic acid, urine oligosaccharide screening and pterins showed all results within normal limits.

Although the repeat lysosomal enzyme analysis was normal, the suspicion was still high for a lysosomal storage disorder largely because of the combined history of a cherry red spot and developmental regression.

Electron microscopy of a skin biopsy (Fig. 1) showed a variety of abnormal inclusions, granular membrane bound vesicles, membrane cytoplasmic bodies (MCB), and zebra bodies. In some cases these were clearly in Schwann cells; in other cases the cell type was unclear. Axons also showed retraction, and debris indicated subacute degeneration. Some axons showed MCB.

Based on this combination of findings, molecular analysis for *GM2A* was considered the next appropriate step. Sequence analysis of *GM2A* did not detect any pathogenic variants; however, despite attempts with multiple primer sets, exon 2 could not be amplified by PCR which suggested a homozygous deletion involving this region. Copy number

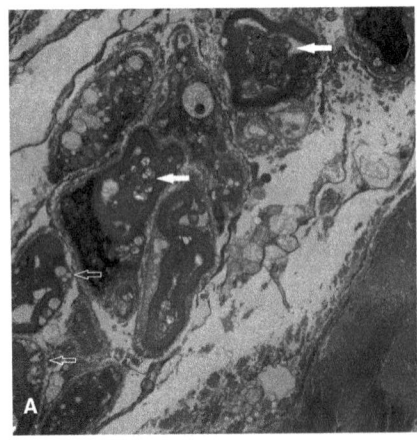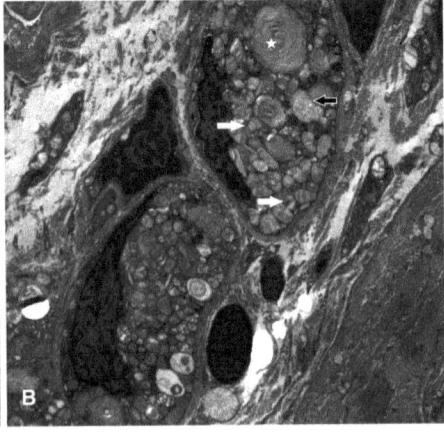

Fig. 1 (**a**) Electron microscopy from a skin biopsy of our patient. Axons with degenerative changes containing membrane bound debris (*solid white arrows*), areas of axonal retraction, and Schwann cell cytoplasm also filled with membrane bound debris (*white outline arrows*). Original magnification 6000x. (**b**) Electron microscopy from a skin biopsy of our patient. Cell with "zebra bodies" (*solid white arrows*), myelinosomes (*white star*), and granular membrane bound vesicles (*outline arrow*). This may represent a Schwann cell but definite myelin is not seen, so identification is uncertain. Original magnification 6000x

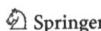

analysis was performed using a custom designed comparative genomic hybridization array, and the child was confirmed to have a homozygous deletion encompassing exon 2 of *GM2A*. Subsequently, breakpoint mapping analysis was performed using PCR amplification and Sanger sequencing, and the genomic breakpoints of the deletion were refined to nucleotide positions g.150,636,648 in intron 1 and g.150,642,789 in intron 2 (Fig. 2). This 6,142 bp deletion has not been previously reported in affected individuals or in the general population. Of note, a 7 bp microhomology was detected at the breakpoint junction.

Discussion

Diagnosis of GM2A deficiency requires the clinician to maintain a high degree of suspicion. In the context of developmental regression, and often a cherry red spot, commonly available biochemical testing (enzyme analysis for both Tay-Sachs disease and Sandhoff disease; urine oligosaccharide screening) will most likely return normal results. Sequence analysis of *HEXA* and *HEXB* may not detect any pathogenic variants. At present, only a small number of cases of GM2A deficiency have been reported worldwide and all reported pathogenic variants are sequence variants that include single nucleotide variants and small (1–3 base pair) deletions that are detectable by sequence analysis (Stenson et al. 2014). The case described herein highlights the need to follow-up in the context of negative biochemical testing, and negative sequence analysis. While our case was homozygous for a whole exon deletion and strongly suspected to be so because of failure of amplification by PCR, an individual with a heterozygous deletion would not have provided the same clue. Moreover, given that only a handful of variants have been associated with disease in the literature, most variants when detected by clinical sequencing would likely be classified as variants of unknown significance (VOUS). As a result, even in a case where a high degree of suspicion leads to the pursuit of sequence

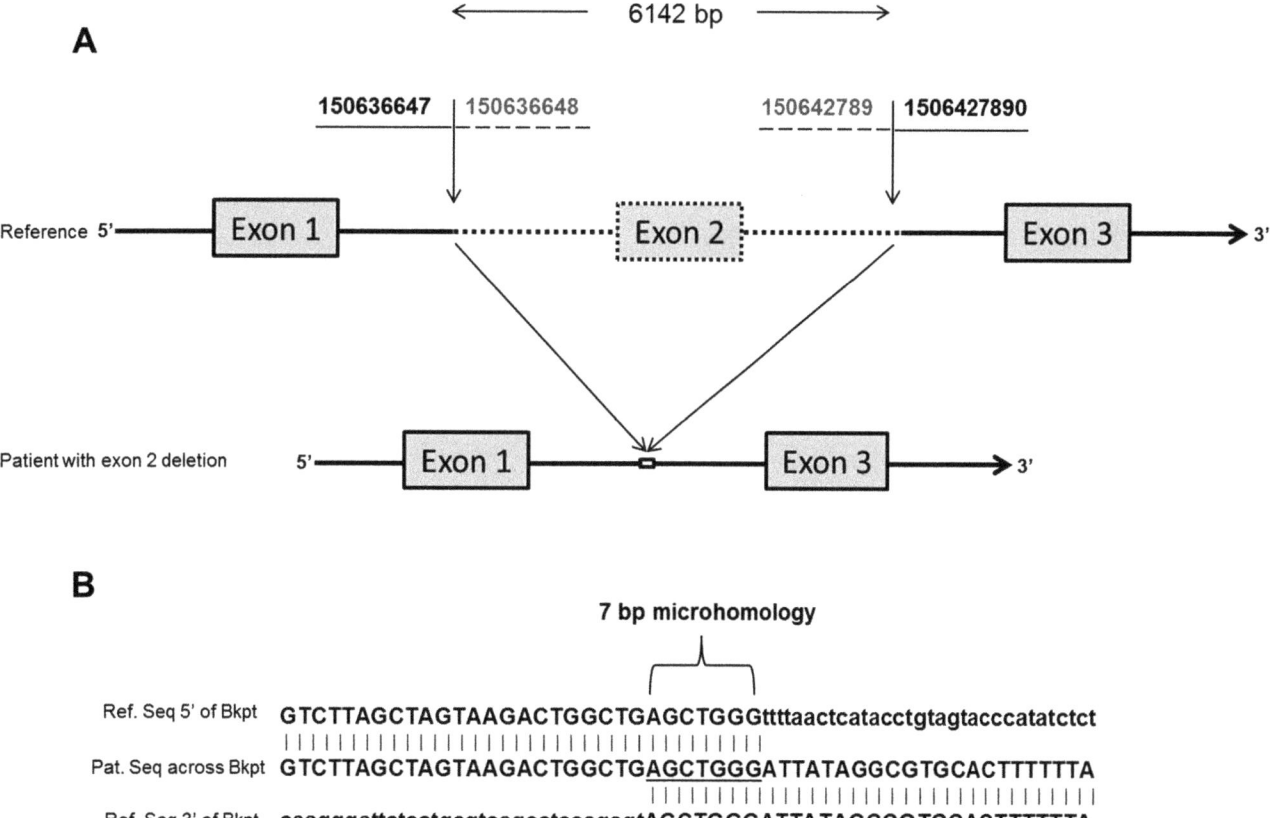

Fig. 2 Exon 2 deletion in *GM2A*. (**a**) Schematic representation of the deletion detected in the *GM2A* gene. The deleted region is represented with *dotted lines* whereas the intact region is represented with *solid lines*. The *downward arrows* indicate the breakpoints of the deletion. Also indicated are the intact (*Black*) and deleted (*Gray*) bases flanking each breakpoint. (**b**) Sequence alignment showing microhomology at the breakpoint junction. Patient sequence across the deletion breakpoint, as obtained by Sanger sequencing, was aligned to the reference sequences from both the 5′ breakpoint and the 3′ breakpoint. As shown in the figure, a 7 bp sequence, "AGCTGGG" was detected on either sides of the deletion. The deletion has been refined to be 6,142 bp long extending from and including chr5:g.150,636,648 to chr5:g.150,642,789. These results, together with the failure of PCR amplification of exon 2, confirm a homozygous deletion of exon 2 of the *GM2A* gene in this individual. *Ref.* reference, *Seq* sequence, *Bkpt* breakpoint

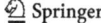

analysis of *GM2A*, a negative result or one in which a single VOUS was detected may end the pursuit without further analysis for larger deletions or duplications.

Our report of the first whole exon deletion expands the spectrum of pathogenic variants identified in the *GM2A* gene and highlights the need for aCGH analysis in the molecular evaluation of GM2A deficiency. In addition, the 7 bp microhomology detected at the breakpoint junction suggests that the deletion may have been mediated by either of the various microhomology-mediated mechanisms that include break-induced serial replication slippage, microhomology mediated break-induced replication, and fork stalling and template switching (Lee et al. 2007; Chen et al. 2010). We also present the first description of electron microscopy findings in GM2 activator deficiency. MCB, lysosomes with granular material, zebra bodies, and myelinosomes are found in the GM2 gangliosidoses and other conditions, including Fabry disease and chloroquine exposure. Myelinosomes have been reported in peripheral ganglia and peripheral nerves in Tay-Sachs disease (Schmitt et al. 1979).

Identification of the precise genetic defect in the proband of any family has several benefits, including putting an end to the diagnostic odyssey, knowing that a treatable disorder was not missed, and enabling the family to pursue advanced reproductive options, such as prenatal diagnosis or preimplantation genetic diagnosis, for future pregnancies. Thorough investigation of the variant spectrum for all diseases will shed light on the need to follow-up negative, or inconclusive sequence results with copy number analysis. In the case of *GM2A*, with the small number of identified cases, and the high degree of clinical suspicion required for the diagnosis, copy number analysis may allow confirmation of additional cases of this rare condition.

Compliance with Ethics Guidelines

Conflict of Interest

Patricia Hall is employed by Emory University and is a laboratory director at EGL Genetic Diagnostics, LLC, a clinical genetics laboratory which performs testing described in this paper.

John Alexander is employed by Emory University and is a laboratory director at EGL Genetic Diagnostics, LLC, a clinical genetics laboratory which performs testing described in this paper.

Arun Ankala is employed by Emory University and is a laboratory director at EGL Genetic Diagnostics, LLC, a clinical genetics laboratory which performs testing described in this paper.

Regina Laine, Hart Lidov, Lisa Teot, and Irina Anselm declare that they have no conflict of interest.

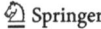

Ethics Approval/Patient Consent

All procedures followed were in accordance with the ethical standards of the responsible committee on human experimentation (institutional and national) and with the Helsinki Declaration of 1975, as revised in 2000 (5). This study was approved by the institutional review boards of Boston Children's Hospital and Emory University where relevant.

Author Contributions

All authors have reviewed and approved the manuscript as submitted.

PLH drafted the manuscript, incorporated edit, reviewed, and interpreted biochemical genetic testing.

RL drafted the clinical synopsis and saw the patient in clinic.

AA and JJA reviewed and interpreted molecular genetic testing.

LAT and HGWL reviewed and interpreted electron microscopy results.

IA saw the patient in clinic and edited the manuscript.

Corresponding Author

Patricia L. Hall, Ph.D.
Department of Human Genetics
Emory University
2165 North Decatur Road
Decatur, GA 30033
patricia.l.hall@emory.edu

Funding

None.

Animal Usage

None.

References

Chen JM, Cooper DN, Ferec C, Kehrer-Sawatzki H, Patrinos GP (2010) Genomic rearrangements in inherited disease and cancer. Semin Cancer Biol 20:222–233

Hall P, Minnich S, Teigen C, Raymond K (2014) Diagnosing lysosomal storage disorders: the GM2 gangliosidoses. Curr Protoc Hum Genet 83:17.16.11–17.16.18

Lee JA, Carvalho CM, Lupski JR (2007) A DNA replication mechanism for generating nonrecurrent rearrangements associated with genomic disorders. Cell 131:1235–1247

Renaud D, Brodsky M (2015) GM2-gangliosidosis, AB variant: clinical, ophthalmological, MRI, and molecular findings. JIMD Rep 25:83–86

Sakuraba H, Itoh K, Shimmoto M et al (1999) GM2 gangliosidosis AB variant: clinical and biochemical studies of a Japanese patient. Neurology 52:372–377

Schepers U, Glombitza G, Lemm T et al (1996) Molecular analysis of a GM2-activator deficiency in two patients with GM2-gangliosidosis AB variant. Am J Hum Genet 59:1048–1056

Schmitt HP, Berlet H, Volk B (1979) Peripheral intraaxonal storage in Tay-Sachs' disease (GM2-gangliosidosis type 1). J Neurol Sci 44:115–124

Schroder M, Schnabel D, Hurwitz R, Young E, Suzuki K, Sandhoff K (1993) Molecular genetics of GM2-gangliosidosis AB variant: a novel mutation and expression in BHK cells. Hum Genet 92:437–440

Smith NJ, Winstone AM, Stellitano L, Cox TM, Verity CM (2012) GM2 gangliosidosis in a UK study of children with progressive neurodegeneration: 73 cases reviewed. Dev Med Child Neurol 54:176–182

Stenson PD, Mort M, Ball EV, Shaw K, Phillips A, Cooper DN (2014) The human gene mutation database: building a comprehensive mutation repository for clinical and molecular genetics, diagnostic testing and personalized genomic medicine. Hum Genet 133:1–9

Xia B, Asif G, Arthur L et al (2013) Oligosaccharide analysis in urine by maldi-tof mass spectrometry for the diagnosis of lysosomal storage diseases. Clin Chem 59:1357–1368

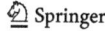

JIMD Reports
DOI 10.1007/8904_2017_32

RESEARCH REPORT

Effect of Lorenzo's Oil on Hepatic Gene Expression and the Serum Fatty Acid Level in *abcd1*-Deficient Mice

**Masashi Morita · Ayako Honda · Akira Kobayashi ·
Yuichi Watanabe · Shiro Watanabe ·
Kosuke Kawaguchi · Shigeo Takashima ·
Nobuyuki Shimozawa · Tsuneo Imanaka**

Received: 12 January 2016 /Revised: 19 April 2017 /Accepted: 2 May 2017 /Published online: 31 May 2017
© SSIEM and Springer-Verlag Berlin Heidelberg 2017

Abstract Lorenzo's oil is known to decrease the saturated very long chain fatty acid (VLCFA) level in the plasma and skin fibroblasts of X-linked adrenoleukodystrophy (ALD) patients. However, the involvement of Lorenzo's oil in in vivo fatty acid metabolism has not been well elucidated. To investigate the effect of Lorenzo's oil on fatty acid metabolism, we analyzed the hepatic gene expression together with the serum fatty acid level in Lorenzo's oil-treated wild-type and *abcd1*-deficient mice. The change in the serum fatty acid level in Lorenzo's oil-treated *abcd1*-defcient mice was quite similar to that in the plasma fatty acid level in ALD patients supplemented with Lorenzo's oil. In addition, we found that the hepatic gene expression of two peroxisomal enzymes, *Dbp* and *Scp2*, and three microsomal enzymes, *Elovl1, 2,* and *3*, were significantly stimulated by Lorenzo's oil. Our findings indicate that Lorenzo's oil activates hepatic peroxisomal fatty acid β-oxidation at the transcriptional level. In contrast, the transcriptional stimulation of *Elovl1, 2,* and *3* by Lorenzo's oil does not cause changes in the serum fatty acid level. It seems likely that the inhibition of these elongation activities by Lorenzo's oil results in a decrease in saturated VLCFA. Thus, these results not only contribute to a clarification of the mechanism by which the saturated VLCFA level is reduced in the serum of ALD patients by Lorenzo's oil-treatment, but also suggest the development of a new therapeutic approach to peroxisomal β-oxidation enzyme deficiency, especially mild phenotype of DBP deficiency.

Communicated by: Robert Steiner

Masashi Morita and Ayako Honda contributed equally to this work.

Electronic supplementary material: The online version of this chapter (doi:10.1007/8904_2017_32) contains supplementary material, which is available to authorized users.

M. Morita (✉) · A. Kobayashi · Y. Watanabe · K. Kawaguchi · T. Imanaka
Department of Biological Chemistry, Graduate School of Medicine and Pharmaceutical Sciences, University of Toyama, 2630 Sugitani, Toyama 930-0194, Japan
e-mail: masa@pha.u-toyama.ac.jp

A. Honda · S. Takashima · N. Shimozawa
Division of Genomic Research, Life Science Research Center, Gifu University, 1-1 Yanagido, Gifu 501-1193, Japan

S. Watanabe
Division of Nutritional Biochemistry, Institute of Natural Medicine, University of Toyama, 2630 Sugitani, Toyama 930-0194, Japan

T. Imanaka
Faculty of Pharmaceutical Sciences, Hiroshima International University, 5-1-1 Hirokoshinkai, Kure, Hiroshima 737-0112, Japan

Introduction

X-linked adrenoleukodystrophy (ALD) (OMIM 300100) is a rare, inherited metabolic disease characterized by an abnormal accumulation of saturated very long chain fatty acids (VLCFAs) such as C24:0 and C26:0 in all tissues (Moser 1997). The abnormal accumulation of lipid molecules containing saturated VLCFAs is thought to be involved in the pathological mechanism underlying ALD. This disease is caused by mutation of the *ABCD1* gene that encodes the peroxisomal ABC protein ABCD1. ABCD1 is a transporter of VLCFA-CoA into peroxisomes (van Roermund et al. 2011). The dysfunction of ABCD1 causes a reduction in peroxisomal VLCFA β-oxidation and an increase in the VLCFA-CoA level in the cytosol (Ofman et al. 2010). The increased cytosolic VLCFA-CoA is used as a substrate for microsomal fatty acid elongation, which results in the accumulation of VLCFAs (Schackmann et al.

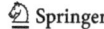

2015). Therefore, lowering the saturated VLCFAs by stimulating peroxisomal fatty acid β-oxidation or by inhibiting microsomal fatty acid elongation is a rational therapeutic approach to ALD.

Until now, two therapeutic approaches have been reportedly investigated: hematopoietic cell transplantation and dietary treatment based on Lorenzo's oil (LO). LO, a 4:1 mixture of glycerol trioleate and glycerol trierucate, is used as a diet supplement to ALD patients (Rizzo et al. 1989). It has been known that LO administration significantly reduces the plasma C26:0 levels in ALD patients (Rizzo et al. 1989; Aubourg et al. 1993; Deon et al. 2008). However, LO does not halt the clinical progression of patients with preexisting neurological dysfunction (Restuccia et al. 1999; Berger and Gartner 2006). On the other hand, it is suggested LO may have a preventative effect in asymptomatic patients (Moser et al. 2005).

Trioleate and trierucate are absorbed from the intestine after being hydrolyzed by lipases and then transported to the liver. Incorporation of erucic acid into the liver was demonstrated in ALD patients who had been administered LO (Murphy et al. 2008). As the bulk of plasma VLCFAs exists as neutral lipids in low density lipoprotein, it is likely that the fatty acid level in plasma is largely associated with lipid metabolism in the liver. We administered LO to both wild-type and *abcd1*-deficient mice, and then analyzed the hepatic gene expression together with the serum level of variety of fatty acids in order to investigate the effect of LO on the hepatic fatty acid metabolism.

Materials and Methods

Mice and Dietary Treatment

The C57BL/6 mice obtained from Clea Japan Inc. and the *abcd1*-deficient mice generated by Kobayashi et al. (1997) were kept at 24 °C ± 2 °C under a dark-light cycle as described previously (Morita et al. 2015). Males aged 4 weeks were used in this experiment. Male C57BL/6 mice and *abcd1*-deficient mice were fed with a powdered chow (CE2, Clea Japan, Inc), supplemented with or without 20% (w/w) LO (SHS International Ltd., Liverpool, UK). All of the mice had free access to food and water. The applied dose of LO was deduced from the daily dose administered to ALD patients as described in De Craemer et al. (1998). The daily intake of LO by the mice on a diet with 20% (w/w) LO was an average of 26 g/kg body weight. After the

treatment, the serum and each tissue were prepared for fatty acid analysis and gene expression analysis and kept at −80 °C before analysis. All of the procedures used in the animal laboratory research were approved by the University Committee for Animal Use and Care at the University of Toyama.

VLCFA Level Analysis

VLCFAs, plasmalogen (C16:0 hexadecanal dimethyl acetal), and phytanic acid in the mouse serum were analyzed as described previously (Takemoto et al. 2003). In screw-capped glass tube, 100 μl of serum were mixed with 2 ml of methanolic hydrochloric acid and the mixture was heated for 2 h at 100 °C. The methyl derivatives were extracted twice with *n*-hexane and subjected to GC/MS system (QP5050A, Shimadzu, Kyoto, Japan), equipped with a capillary INNOWAX column (Hewlett-Packard, Palo Alto, CA, USA) and an autosampler/autoinjector (AOC-20, Shimazu). The fatty acid analysis in liver was also performed as described previously (Morita et al. 2015).

Quantitative Real-Time PCR

After the mice were sacrificed, the livers and brains were removed and quickly frozen in lipid N_2. Total RNA was purified with Isogen (Nippon Gene, Japan) and cDNA was synthesized with M-MLV reverse transcriptase (Invitrogen, CA). Gene expression analysis was performed with fluorescent Taqman methodology, using the StepOnePlus™ Real-Time PCR System (Applied Biosystems, CA). Real-time quantitative PCR was performed for each of the following genes, using ready-to use primer and probe sets pre-developed by Applied Biosystems (TaqMan gene expression assays): *Acox1* (Mm00443579_m1), acetyl-Coenzyme A acyltransferase 1A (*Acaa1a*, Mm00728460_s1), *Dbp* (Mm0050043_m1), *Scp2* (Mm01257982_m1), *Abcd2* (Mm00496455_m1), *Pparα-1 and 2* (Mm00627559_m1 for boundary between exon 3 and 4, and Mm00440939_ml for 7 and 8, respectively), *Elovl1* (Mm00517077_m1), *Elovl2* (Mm00517086_m1), *Elovl3* (Mm00468164_m1), *Elovl4* (Mm00521704_m1), *Elovl5* (Mm00506717_m1), *Elovl6* (Mm00851223_s1), and *Gapdh* (Hs99999905_m1) as an endogenous control. The mRNA Ct values for these genes were normalized to *Gapdh* and expressed as a relative increase or decrease in the tissues from the non-treated mice to those in the LO-treated mice.

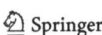

Statistical Analysis

Statistical analysis was performed with unpaired t-test, using the Bonferroni correction for multiple comparisons.

Results and Discussion

Administration of LO to Wild-Type and *abcd1*-Deficient Mice

Wild-type or *abcd1*-deficent 4-week-old mice were fed a diet containing LO for 5 weeks. The average consumptions of laboratory chow in wild-type mice with or without LO were 2.45 g/day and 2.80 g/day, respectively. The average consumptions were 2.50 g/day and 2.87 g/day in *abcd1*-deficient mice with or without LO, respectively. From the intake of diet, the mice were fed approximately 26 g of LO per kg of body weight daily. This almost corresponds to the treatment of LO for ALD therapy in patients. The intake of LO had no effect on body weight in either the wild-type or *abcd1*-deficient mice (Supplementary Fig. 1). After 5 weeks, the serum fatty acid level and hepatic gene expression were analyzed.

Changes in Fatty Acid Level in Serum from LO-Treated Mice

We previously reported that a high-fat diet consisting mainly of C16:0, C18:1, and C18:2 activates hepatic peroxisomal VLCFA metabolism (Kozawa et al. 2011). To date, however, the effect of LO on hepatic fatty acid metabolism has not been reported. In the present study, we first analyzed the fatty acid level in the serum from wild-type and *abcd1*-deficient mice fed a diet with or without LO. In *abcd1*-deficient mice, the level of saturated VLCFAs such as C20:0, C22:0, C24:0, and C26:0 was higher than those in the wild-type mice. In particular, the level of C26:0 in *abcd1*-deficient mice was nearly four times higher than that in the wild-type mice. As a result of treatment with LO, the concentration (μg/100 μl serum) of C26:0 and the ratio of C26:0/C22:0 were decreased to a level similar to that in wild-type mice (Table 1 and Fig. 1). These results clearly indicate that LO has the capacity to reduce the saturated

Table 1 Effect of Lorenzo's oil on the level of serum fatty acids

Fatty acid	WT	WT + LO	KO	KO + LO
C14:0	0.643 ± 0.082	0.378 ± 0.015	0.941 ± 0.061	$0.375 \pm 0.007^{***}$
C14:1	0.018 ± 0.008	0.004 ± 0.001	0.033 ± 0.006	$0.005 \pm 0.001^{*}$
C16:0DMA	0.897 ± 0.059	0.769 ± 0.026	0.920 ± 0.027	0.883 ± 0.040
C16:0	29.96 ± 1.674	24.62 ± 0.982	$41.01 \pm 0.834^{\#\#\#}$	$26.70 \pm 1.047^{**}$
C16:1	3.986 ± 0.763	0.904 ± 0.102	7.580 ± 0.502	$0.995 \pm 0.083^{***}$
Phytanic acid	0.443 ± 0.037	$0.255 \pm 0.009^{**}$	0.515 ± 0.018	$0.258 \pm 0.013^{***}$
C18:0	12.02 ± 0.207	$16.01 \pm 0.399^{***}$	$13.76 \pm 0.239^{\#}$	16.07 ± 0.763
C18:1	26.42 ± 2.652	$48.83 \pm 3.745^{*}$	34.95 ± 0.438	$48.87 \pm 3.003^{*}$
C18:2	39.77 ± 1.267	33.59 ± 0.893	$47.68 \pm 1.034^{\#}$	$35.46 \pm 0.867^{***}$
C18:3	1.142 ± 0.136	$0.378 \pm 0.048^{*}$	$1.952 \pm 0.113^{\#}$	$0.366 \pm 0.043^{***}$
C20:0	0.325 ± 0.023	0.334 ± 0.037	$0.615 \pm 0.009^{\#\#\#}$	$0.394 \pm 0.038^{*}$
C20:1	0.844 ± 0.141	$2.300 \pm 0.111^{***}$	1.356 ± 0.052	1.889 ± 0.139
C20:4 (ARA)	5.039 ± 0.187	$8.483 \pm 0.465^{***}$	5.891 ± 0.162	$8.991 \pm 0.206^{***}$
C20:5 (EPA)	5.069 ± 0.178	$3.417 \pm 0.146^{***}$	$7.095 \pm 0.112^{\#\#\#}$	$3.772 \pm 0.170^{***}$
C22:0	0.530 ± 0.014	$0.314 \pm 0.044^{*}$	$0.646 \pm 0.013^{\#\#}$	$0.461 \pm 0.031^{*}$
C22:1	0.126 ± 0.024	$2.852 \pm 0.497^{*}$	$0.255 \pm 0.005^{\#}$	3.297 ± 0.715
C24:0	0.386 ± 0.023	$0.126 \pm 0.014^{***}$	$0.544 \pm 0.004^{\#\#\#}$	$0.202 \pm 0.011^{***}$
C24:1	1.455 ± 0.083	$3.877 \pm 0.061^{***}$	1.211 ± 0.027	$4.232 \pm 0.128^{***}$
C22:6 (DHA)	19.05 ± 0.484	$15.84 \pm 0.321^{*}$	19.24 ± 0.983	16.90 ± 0.679
C25:0	0.010 ± 0.001	0.005 ± 0.000	0.021 ± 0.003	0.009 ± 0.000
C26:0	0.008 ± 0.001	0.005 ± 0.001	$0.033 \pm 0.002^{\#\#\#}$	$0.010 \pm 0.001^{***}$

Wild-type (WT) ($n = 4$) and *abcd1*-deficient (KO) mice ($n = 4$) were fed with (+LO) or without LO for 5 weeks, as in Supplementary Fig. 1. The serum was prepared from each mouse and subjected to gas chromatography/mass spectrometry (GC/MS) analysis. Values are expressed as μg fatty acid/100 μl serum and are the mean $\pm$ S.E. for 4 determinations. Where "*" is indicated, the values for LO-treated mice are significantly different from non-treated mice, $^{*} <0.02$, $^{**} <0.005$, $^{***} <0.002$. Where "#" is indicated, the values for *abcd1*-deficient mice were significantly different from wild-type mice, $^{\#} <0.02$, $^{\#\#} <0.005$, $^{\#\#\#} <0.002$. Statistical analysis was analyzed by unpaired t-test, using the Bonferroni correction for multiple comparisons

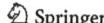

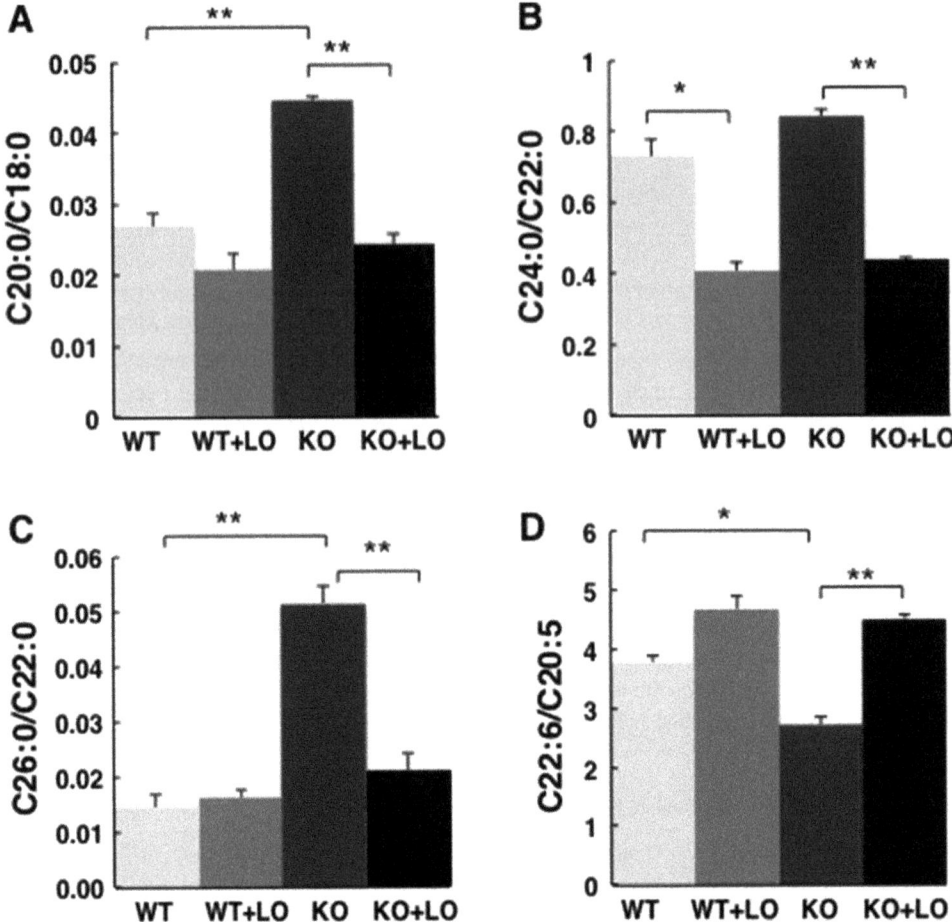

Fig. 1 Serum fatty acids level in LO-treated mice. The ratios of C20:0/C18:0 (**a**), C24:0/C20:0 (**b**), C26:0/C22:0 (**c**), and C22:6/C20:5 (**d**) calculated from Table 1 are shown. The values are the mean ± S.

E. ($n = 4$ animals. *, $p < 0.005$, **, $p < 0.002$). Statistical analysis was performed with unpaired t-test, using the Bonferroni correction for multiple comparisons

VLCFA level in serum of *abcd1*-deficient mice. This is consistent with reports that the C26:0 level in plasma from ALD patients was decreased to a normal level by 4-week-treatment with LO (Rizzo et al. 1989). In addition, as reported in LO-treated ALD patients (Moser et al. 1999), an increase of the mono-unsaturated fatty acids such as C18:1, C20:1, C22:1, and C24:1 along with a decrease of n-3 polyunsaturated fatty acids such as linolenic acid (C18:3n-3) and eicosapentanoic acid (EPA) (C20:5n-3) were also observed in the LO-treated *abcd1*-deficient mice. These results indicate that the effect of LO on the fatty acid metabolism was quite similar in *abcd1*-deficient mice and ALD patients.

EPA (C20:5n-3) is known to be converted sequentially to C22:5, C24:5, C24:6 and then DHA (C22:6n-3) via fatty acid elongation, desaturation, and β-oxidation, respectively (Ferdinandusse et al. 2001). As the final β-oxidation is a limiting step in the peroxisome, the C24:6/C22:6 ratio is a

reliable measure of the impairment of peroxisomal β-oxidation. In addition, the C26:1 level is reported to be elevated in the insufficiency of peroxisomal β-oxidation (Fourcade et al. 2010). However, C26:1 as well as the intermediate fatty acids such as C22:5, C24:5, and C24:6 during the synthesis of C22:6 from C20:5 could not be detected in our assay system using GC/MS (Takemoto et al. 2003). Therefore, we showed C22:6/C20:5 ratio as a marker of peroxisomal fatty acid β-oxidation in this study (Fig. 1). As shown, C22:6/C20:5 ratio in *abcd1*-deficient mice was lower than in wild-type mice, but was significantly increased by LO, suggesting that peroxisomal β-oxidation in *abcd1*-defcient mice may be partly recovered. Peroxisomal VLCFA β-oxidation consists of the ABCD1-dependent and -independent pathways (Morita et al. 2012). In *abcd1*-deficient mice, LO seems to stimulate the latter pathway in which VLCFA-CoA is imported into peroxisomes by functionally related homologs, ABCD2 or

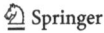

ABCD3, or VLCFA is diffused through the lipid barrier and activated to VLCFA-CoA by very long chain acyl-CoA synthetases, such as ACSVL1 and ACSVL5. In contrast to the ratio of C22:6/C20:5, the ratios of C20:0/C18:0 and C24:0/C22:0 were largely decreased in LO-treated wild-type and *abcd1*-deficient mice (Fig. 1), suggesting that the elongation of C18:0 and C22:0 to C20:0 and C24:0 may be depressed by LO treatment. It is therefore possible that the level of saturated VLCFAs was decreased by either activating peroxisomal fatty acid β-oxidation or by inhibiting microsomal fatty acid elongation. Further detailed analyses for the other markers representing the above fatty acid metabolic systems are believed to provide a complete view of the efficacies of LO.

In mice, the level of phytanic acid and palmitoleic acid (C16:1) is decreased and the level of arachidonic acid (C20:4) is increased by LO treatment, which is different from result in ALD patients supplemented with LO (Moser et al. 1999).

Changes in Hepatic Gene Expression in LO-Treated Mice

As the fatty acid level in serum is thought to be affected by the fatty acid metabolism in the liver, we next analyzed the effect of LO on hepatic gene expression in both wild-type and *abcd1*-deficient mice. The level of C26:0 in the liver from *abcd1*-deficient mice (6.0 ± 0.5 μg/g tissue weight) was higher than that from wild-type mice (1.3 ± 0.2 μg/g

tissue weight). However, the level was significantly decreased (4.0 ± 0.1 μg/g tissue weight) in LO-treated *abcd1*-defcient mice (Supplementary Fig. 2). Figure 2 shows the gene expression of the representative enzymes that are involved in peroxisomal fatty acid β-oxidation and microsomal fatty acid elongation. *Abcd2* gene encodes ABCD2 protein. *Acox1* and *Acaa1a* genes encode an acyl-CoA oxidase protein and a straight-chain 3-oxo-acyl thiolase, respectively. *Dbp* gene encodes D-bifunctional protein that has enoyl-CoA hydratase and 3-hydroxyacyl-CoA dehydrogenase activities, and generates 3-ketoacyl-CoAs (Ferdinandusse et al. 2006a). *Scp2* gene encodes SCPx, a peroxisome-associated thiolase, which involved in the oxidation of branched-chain fatty acids (Seedorf et al. 1994; Ferdinandusse et al. 2006b). *Elovl* genes encode enzymes responsible for the first and rate-limiting step of fatty acid elongation reaction in ER. In contrast, *Ppara* gene encodes PPARα, a transcription factor and a major regulator of lipid metabolism in the liver. The mRNA expression of these genes was almost the same in the wild-type and *abcd1*-deficient mice fed by normal diet (Fig. 2) although the expression of *Ppara* in the *abcd1*-deficient mice was higher, but not significantly, compared with wild-type mice. When wild or *abcd1*-deficient mice were administered with LO, the gene expression of *Dbp*, *Scp2*, *Elovl1, 2, 3, and 5* was significantly increased in both the wild-type and *abcd1*-deficient mice. The expression of *Abcd2* and *Ppara* was also increased by the treatment with

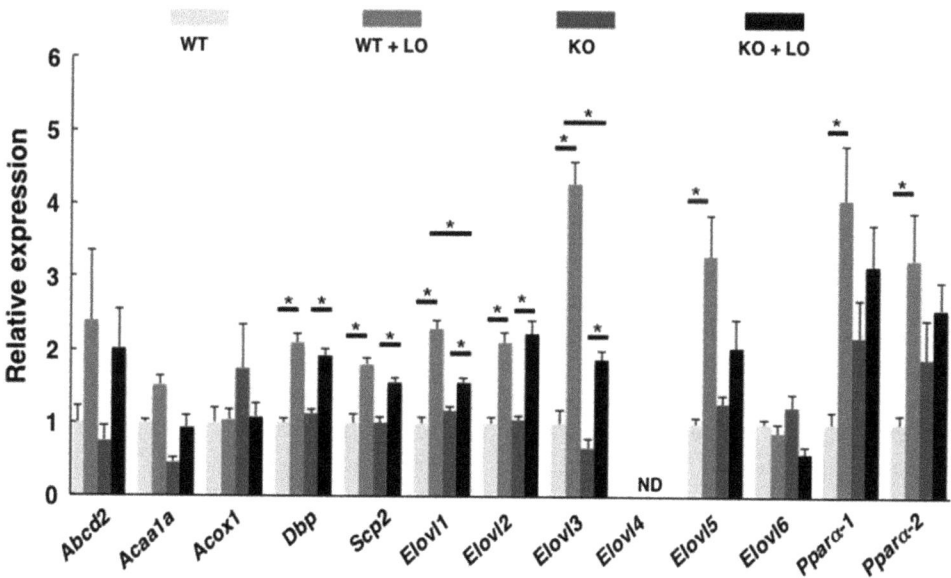

Fig. 2 Gene expression profiles in LO-treated mice liver. The relative gene expressions of liver from wild-type (WT) or *abcd1*-deficient (KO) mice with or without LO were analyzed by real-time PCR. *Ppara-1* and *Ppara-2* are genes detected by probes for recognizing distinct position of *Ppara* sequence. The gene expression of *Elovl4* gene was not detected (ND). Values are mean ± S.E. (*n* = 4 animals. *, *p* < 0.05)

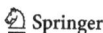

LO in both the wild-type and *abcd1*-deficient mice, although there was no significant difference in *abcd1*-deficient mice. The up-regulation of *Abcd2, Dbp, Scp2,* and *Pparα* gene indicates that LO has the capacity to activate hepatic peroxisomal fatty acid β-oxidation, which may thereby participate in the decrease of saturated VLCFA. This is consistent with the reports that show high-fat diets rich in erucic acid induced hepatic peroxisomal fatty acid β-oxidation in rodents (Neat et al. 1981; Bremer and Norum 1982; Thomassen et al. 1985; Veerkamp and Zevenbergen 1986). As DBP and SCPx are involved in the peroxisomal β-oxidation of branched-chain fatty acids and bile acid intermediates (Seedorf et al. 1994; Ferdinandusse et al. 2006a, b), LO might exert an effect on the β-oxidation of not only saturated VLCFAs, but also branched-chain fatty acids or bile acid intermediates, in peroxisomes.

In microsomal fatty acid elongation reactions, the ELOVLs are responsible for the first and rate-limiting steps in the reaction cycle (Jump 2009). Among them, ELOVL1 and 3, encoded by *ELOVL1* and *3*, respectively, are involved in the synthesis of saturated and mono-unsaturated fatty acids (Sassa and Kihara 2014). In contrast, ELOVL2 and 5, encoded by *ELOVL2* and *5*, respectively, are involved in poly-unsaturated fatty acid metabolism. In ALD, ELOVL1 is thought to mainly be involved in the accumulation of saturated VLCFAs, because the accumulation of C26:0 was decreased by a silencing of the *ELOVL1* gene in ALD fibroblasts (Ofman et al. 2010). However, the hepatic gene expression of *Elovls* was the same in the wild-type and *abcd1*-deficient mice. In addition, we found that the *Elovl1* and *3* genes were quite stimulated by the treatment with LO, while the level of C26:0 was decreased (Table 1 and Supplementary Fig. 2). These results indicate that the decrease of saturated VLCFAs by LO was not regulated at the transcriptional level. Recently, Sassa et al. reported that in an in vitro experiment LO reduced the synthesis of saturated VLCFAs by inhibiting ELOVL1 at the protein but not transcriptional level (Sassa et al. 2014). The elongations of both C18:0 to C20:0 and C22:0 to C24:0, which are catalyzed by ELOVL1 and 3, appear to be largely inhibited by the treatment with LO. Therefore, we speculated that LO suppressed these fatty acid elongation activities, which resulted in a decrease in saturated VLCFAs. The decrease in the saturated VLCFA level can stimulate *Elovl1* and *3* genes expression. It has been reported that *Elovl3* expression is elevated in mice lacking the ABCD2 protein that is involved in the peroxisomal β-oxidation of monounsaturated VLCFA (Brolinson et al. 2008). In LO-treated mice, the gene expression of *Elovl1* and *Elovl3* in the *abcd1*-deficient mice was lower than that in wild-type mice. It is therefore possible that the *Elovl1*

and *3* gene expression is tightly regulated by the level of mono-unsaturated and saturated VLCFAs.

In LO-treated mice, the level of n-3 polyunsaturated VLCFA (C20:5 and C22:6) was decreased (Table 1). As the synthesis of n-3 polyunsaturated VLCFAs is known to be mediated by ELOVL2 and 5, it seems likely that the decrease of n-3 polyunsaturated VLCFAs was, at least in part, due to the inhibition of ELOVL2 and 5 activities by LO.

In the present study, we found that effect of LO on the serum fatty acid level in *abcd1*-deficient mice was quite similar to that on the plasma fatty acid level in ALD patients as reported by Moser et al. (1999). Therefore, *abcd1*-deficient mice are useful for investigating the effect of LO on in vivo fatty acid metabolism. In the present study, we first reported that LO has remarkable effects on the hepatic gene expression involved in peroxisomal fatty acid β-oxidation and microsomal fatty acid elongation. More recently, van Engen et al. showed that mutation of Cyp4f2 decreases the conversion of VLCFA into very long chain dicarboxylic acids by ω-oxidation (van Engen et al. 2016). As the ω-oxidation is a potential escape route for the deficient peroxisomal VLCFA β-oxidation in ALD, it is interesting whether LO induces expression of *Cyp4f2* gene.

Much less is known about the relevance of these findings in mice for human physiology. Nonetheless, our results can help provide novel insights into the metabolic impact of LO on in vivo fatty acid metabolism. Furthermore, we found that the hepatic gene expression of *Dbp* was increased by LO-treatment in both the wild-type and *abcd1*-deficient mice, which suggests that LO-treatment may be a candidate therapy for DBP deficiency. DBP deficiency has been classified into 3 subgroups (Wanders et al. 2001) and recently, several patients with a less severe form of DBP have been reported by whole-exome sequencing (PMID: 27790638). Mutant DBP in patients with less severe form seems to possess some degree of enzyme activity. Our results suggest that LO may have a capacity to increase hepatic *DBP* gene expression as well as decrease serum saturated VLCFAs in DBP patients. Further investigation is required, not only studies using *dbp*-deficient mice but also clinical research for patients with mild phenotype of DBP deficiency.

Acknowledgements We thank Akiko Ohba, Kayoko Toyoshi, and Noritake Taniguchi for technical assistance. This research was supported in part by a Grant-in-Aid for Scientific Research from the Ministry of Education, Culture, Sports, Science and Technology of Japan (16K09961, 15H04875, 15K15389). Pacific Edit reviewed the manuscript prior to submission.

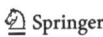

Take-Home Message

Lorenzo's oil activates hepatic peroxisomal fatty acid β-oxidation at the transcriptional level.

Conflict of Interest

Masashi Morita, Ayako Honda, Akira Kobayashi, Yuichi Watanabe, Shiro Watanabe, Kosuke Kawaguchi, Shigeo Takashima, Nobuyuki Shimozawa, and Tsuneo Imanaka declare that they have no conflict of interest.

Informed Consent

This article does not contain any studies with human participants performed by any of the authors.

Animal Rights

All institutional and national guidelines for the care and use of laboratory animals were followed. All procedures performed in studies involving animals were in accordance with the ethical standards of the University Committee for Animal Use and Care at the University of Toyama.

Author Contributions

TI conceived and supervised the study; TI, MM, AH, and NS designed experiments; MM, AH, AK, YW, KK, ST, and SW performed the experiments; MM, TI, and NS wrote the manuscript, which was discussed by all authors.

References

Aubourg P, Adamsbaum C, Lavallard-Rousseau MC et al (1993) A two-year trial of oleic and erucic acids ("Lorenzo's oil") as treatment for adrenomyeloneuropathy. N Engl J Med 329:745–752

Berger J, Gartner J (2006) X-linked adrenoleukodystrophy: clinical, biochemical and pathogenetic aspects. Biochim Biophys Acta 1763:1721–1732

Bremer J, Norum KR (1982) Metabolism of very long-chain monounsaturated fatty acids (22:1) and the adaptation to their presence in the diet. J Lipid Res 23:243–256

Brolinson A, Fourcade S, Jakobsson A, Pujol A, Jacobsson A (2008) Steroid hormones control circadian Elovl3 expression in mouse liver. Endocrinology 149:3158–3166

De Craemer D, Van den Branden C, Fontaine M, Vamecq J (1998) Effects of Lorenzo's oil on peroxisomes in healthy mice. Prostaglandins Other Lipid Mediat 55:237–244

Deon M, Garcia MP, Sitta A et al (2008) Hexacosanoic and docosanoic acids plasma levels in patients with cerebral childhood and asymptomatic X-linked adrenoleukodystrophy: Lorenzo's oil effect. Metac Brain Dis 23:43–49

Ferdinandusse S, Denis S, Mooijer PA et al (2001) Identification of the peroxisomal β-oxidation enzymes involved in the biosynthesis of docosahexaenoic acid. J Lipid Res 42:1987–1995

Ferdinandusse S, Denis S, Mooyer PA et al (2006a) Clinical and biochemical spectrum of D-bifunctional protein deficiency. Ann Neurol 59:92–104

Ferdinandusse S, Kostopoulos P, Denis S et al (2006b) Mutations in the gene encoding peroxisomal sterol carrier protein X (SCPx) cause leukencephalopathy with dystonia and motor neuropathy. Am J Hum Genet 78:1046–1052

Fourcade S, Ruiz M, Guilera C et al (2010) Valproic acid induces antioxidant effects in X-linked adrenoleukodystrophy. Hum Mol Genet 19:2005–2014

Jump DB (2009) Mammalian fatty acid elongases. Methods Mol Biol 579:375–389

Kobayashi T, Shinnoh N, Kondo A, Yamada T (1997) Adrenoleukodystrophy protein-deficient mice represent abnormality of very long chain fatty acid metabolism. Biochem Biophys Res Commun 232:631–636

Kozawa S, Honda A, Kajiwara N et al (2011) Induction of peroxisomal lipid metabolism in mice fed a high-fat diet. Mol Med Rep 4:1157–1162

Morita M, Kawamichi M, Shimura Y, Kawaguchi K, Watanabe S, Imanaka T (2015) Brain microsomal fatty acid elongation is increased in abcd1-deficient mouse during active myelination phase. Metab Brain Dis 30:1359–1367

Morita M, Shinbo S, Asahi A, Imanaka T (2012) Very long chain fatty acid β-oxidation in astrocytes: contribution of the ABCD1-dependent and -independent pathways. Biol Pharm Bull 35:1972–1979

Moser AB, Jones DS, Raymond GV, Moser HW (1999) Plasma and red blood cell fatty acids in peroxisomal disorders. Neurochem Res 24:187–197

Moser HW (1997) Adrenoleukodystrophy: phenotype, genetics, pathogenesis and therapy. Brain 120:1485–1508

Moser HW, Raymond GV, Lu SE et al (2005) Follow-up of 89 asymptomatic patients with adrenoleukodystrophy treated with Lorenzo's oil. Arch Neurol 62:1073–1080

Murphy CC, Murphy EJ, Golovko MY (2008) Erucic acid is differentially taken up and metabolized in rat liver and heart. Lipids 43:391–400

Neat CE, Thomassen MS, Osmundsen H (1981) Effects of high-fat diets on hepatic fatty acid oxidation in the rat. Isolation of rat liver peroxisomes by vertical-rotor centrifugation by using a self-generated, iso-osmotic, Percoll gradient. Biochem J 196:149–159

Ofman R, Dijkstra IM, van Roermund CW (2010) The role of ELOVL1 in very long-chain fatty acid homeostasis and X-linked adrenoleukodystrophy. EMBO Mol Med 2:90–97

Restuccia D, Di Lazzaro V, Valeriani M et al (1999) Neurophysiologic follow-up of long-term dietary treatment in adult-onset adrenoleukodystrophy. Neurology 52:810–816

Rizzo WB, Leshner RT, Odone A et al (1989) Dietary erucic acid therapy for X-linked adrenoleukodystrophy. Neurology 39:1415–1422

Sassa T, Kihara A (2014) Metabolism of very-long-chain fatty acids: genes and pathophysiology. Biomol Ther 22:83–92

Sassa T, Wakashima T, Ohno Y, Kihara A (2014) Lorenzo's oil inhibits ELOVL1 and lowers the level of sphingomyelin with a saturated very-long-chain fatty acid. J Lipid Res 55:524–530

Schackmann MJ, Ofman R, Dijkstra IM, Wanders RJ, Kemp S (2015) Enzymatic characterization of ELOVL1, a key enzyme in very long-chain fatty acid synthesis. Biochim Biophys Acta 1851:231–237

Seedorf U, Brysch P, Engel T, Schrage K, Assmann G (1994) Sterol carrier protein X is peroxisomal 3-oxoacyl coenzyme a thiolase with intrinsic sterol carrier and lipid transfer activity. J Biol Chem 269:21277–21283

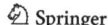

Takemoto Y, Suzuki Y, Horibe R, Shimozawa N, Wanders RJ, Kondo N (2003) Gas chromatography/mass spectrometry analysis of very long chain fatty acids, docosahexaenoic acid, phytanic acid and plasmalogen for the screening of peroxisomal disorders. Brain Dev 25:481–487

Thomassen MS, Norseth J, Christiansen EN (1985) Long-term effects of high-fat diets on peroxisomal β-oxidation in male and female rats. Lipids 20:668–674

van Engen CE, Ofman R, Dijkstra IM et al (2016) CYP4F2 affects phenotypic outcome in adrenoleukodystrophy by modulating the clearance of very long-chain fatty acids. Biochim Biophys Acta 1862:1861–1870

van Roermund CW, Visser WF, Ijlst L, Waterham HR, Wanders RJ (2011) Differential substrate specificities of human ABCD1 and ABCD2 in peroxisomal fatty acid β-oxidation. Biochim Biophys Acta 1811:148–152

Veerkamp JH, Zevenbergen JL (1986) Effect of dietary fat on total and peroxisomal fatty acid oxidation in rat tissues. Biochim Biophys Acta 878:102–109

Wanders RJA, Barth PG, Heymans HAS (2001) Single peroxisomal enzyme deficiencies. In: Scriver CR, Beaudet AL, Sly WS, Valle D (eds) The molecular and metabolic basis of inherited disease. McGraw-Hill, New York, pp 3219–3256

JIMD Reports
DOI 10.1007/8904_2017_33

RESEARCH REPORT

Introduction of a Simple Second Tier Screening Test for C5 Isobars in Dried Blood Spots: Reducing the False Positive Rate for Isovaleric Acidaemia in Expanded Newborn Screening

R. S. Carling · D. Burden · I. Hutton · R. Randle · K. John · J. R. Bonham

Received: 21 April 2017 / Revised: 27 May 2017 / Accepted: 30 May 2017 / Published online: 20 June 2017
© SSIEM and Springer-Verlag Berlin Heidelberg 2017

Abstract In 2015 the English Newborn Screening programme expanded to include Isovaleric Acidaemia (IVA). Screening is performed by flow injection analysis tandem mass spectrometry of isovalerylcarnitine. Isovalerylcarnitine is isobaric with pivaloylcarnitine which can be present in blood due to the use of pivalic ester pro-drugs or pivalic acid derivatives used as emollients in some nipple creams; the potential for false positives (FP) is well documented. A pilot study in England screened 438,164 babies, 18 had presumptive positive results but only 4 were confirmed as true positives (TP). We developed a simple test to separate the isobaric compounds and investigate these samples further.

We studied newborn screening blood spots from 122 randomised controls and 34 infants with an initial raised C5 result. Dried blood spots were eluted with 30% acetonitrile (150 µL) and injected into a Waters Acquity UPLC coupled to a Waters Premier XE tandem mass spectrometer operating in positive ion mode. Isocratic separation of isovalerylcarnitine, pivaloylcarnitine, valerylcarnitine and 2-methylbutyrylcarnitine was achieved within 8 min. Assay performance characteristics were acceptable and non-parametric reference ranges ($n = 122$) were determined for each analyte.

If this method had been used as a second tier test for the 34 presumptive positive samples, the number of FP's would have reduced from 24 to 8 and the positive predictive value of the screening test would have increased from 29 to 56%. Introduction of this test into the screening protocol has the potential to significantly reduce FP results for IVA and prevent unnecessary anxiety.

Introduction

Isovaleric acidaemia (IVA) is an autosomal recessive disorder of leucine metabolism, with an estimated prevalence of 1 in 123,457 in western populations (Moorthie et al. 2013). The phenotypic abnormalities seen in IVA are due to the accumulation of isovaleric acid, which is toxic to the central nervous system and it is the excess 3-hydroxyisovaleric acid which is responsible for the unusual "sweaty foot" odour associated with these patients during an acute episode.

IVA can present as one of three forms, acute neonatal, chronic intermittent (Tanaka 1990; Vockley et al. 1992) or the more recently recognised milder phenotype (Ensenauer et al. 2004). The biochemical diagnosis of IVA is based upon an abnormal acylcarnitine profile, with a prominent increase in isovalerylcarnitine, and a urine organic acid profile with increased excretion of 3-hydroxyisovaleric acid and isovalerylglycine. IsovalerylCoA dehydrogenase (IVD) activity can also be measured in fibroblasts and lymphocytes if required. More than 25 mutations in the IVD gene have been described, some of which result in complete absence of the enzyme. Recent evidence indicates that the 932C > T (A282V) IVD mutation is associated with a

Communicated by: Bridget Wilcken

R. S. Carling (✉) · D. Burden · I. Hutton · R. Randle · K. John
South East Thames Regional Newborn Screening Laboratory,
Biochemical Sciences, Viapath, Guys & St Thomas' NHSFT, 4th
Floor, North Wing, Westminster Bridge Road, London SE1 7EH, UK
e-mail: rachel.carling@viapath.co.uk

J. R. Bonham
Division of Pharmacy, Diagnostics and Genetics, Sheffield Children's
(NHS) FT, Sheffield, UK

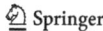

milder phenotype whereas heterogeneous IVD gene mutations tend to correlate with more severe disease (Ensenauer et al. 2004).

In recent years, IVA has been added to newborn screening programs in many centres across Europe, America and Australasia. IVA is a good candidate for newborn screening; there is a simple and acceptable screening test available and ready access to confirmatory testing. The characteristic presentation of acute IVA is in the first 2 weeks of life and if left untreated, IVA is associated with approximately 50% mortality rate and there is a likelihood of severe neurological symptoms and learning disability.

Newborn screening for IVA is based on flow injection analysis tandem mass spectrometry of isovalerylcarnitine. Isovalerylcarnitine is isobaric with pivaloylcarnitine which can be present in blood due to maternal use of pivalic ester pro-drugs or pivalic acid derivatives used as emollients in some nipple creams; the potential for FP results is well documented. Abdenur et al. (1998) first reported a FP newborn screening result on a baby whose mother was taking pivaloyl containing antibiotics. Further investigation of a urine sample by Gas Chromatography Mass Spectrometry revealed the presence of methylpivaloate and the pivaloylcarnitine was shown to decrease once the antibiotics were withdrawn. Common examples of such drugs include Pivmecillinam, the pivaloyloxymethyl ester of Mecillinam and Pivampicillin, the pivaloylmethyl ester of Ampicillin. Boemer et al. (2014) reported 50 FP IVA results detected in Belgium during an 18-month period which were subsequently investigated and found to be due to the use of a nipple fissure ungent containing pivallic acid derivatives. This particular nipple cream was routinely supplied to breastfeeding mothers in a specific hospital and correlated with an increase in the number of positive results from 0.2 to 1.4% over an 18-month period. The pivalate derivative acts as an emollient and is absorbed from the nipple cream by the baby during breastfeeding. In the UK, many nipple fissure ungents are based on lanolin and do not appear to contain pivalic acid derivatives, however, at least one product has been identified as containing pivaloyl derivatives (described as "neopentanoate" or "isodecylneopentanoate"). This was "Mustela Nursing Comfort Balm" and was being used by at least one of the mothers of the FP IVA babies described here. Boemer et al. (2014) successfully developed an LCMSMS method to separate the isovalerylcarnitine from its isobars. However, this method was based on derivatisation of the blood spot extract prior to analysis making it less suitable to rapid turnaround. The method described here is simple and does not require derivatisation of the blood spot prior to analysis making it suitable for inclusion as a second tier screening test. In the event of a screen positive sample being detected, isobar analysis could be rapidly performed ensuring that there was minimal delay in clinical referral of a TP sample.

Materials and Methods

Isovaleryl-L-carnitine and Tridecafluoroheptanoic acid were purchased from Sigma Aldrich. Pivaloyl-L-carnitine hydrochloride, valeryl-L-carnitine hydrochloride and 2-methylbutyryl-L-carnitine hydrochloride were purchased from VU University Medical centre, Amsterdam. [^{2}H$_9$]-isovalerylcarnitine was purchased from CDN Isotopes. A stock standard containing 10 mM isovalerylcarnitine, pivaloylcarnitine, valerylcarnitine and 2-methylbutyrylcarnitine in 100% methanol was prepared. This was used to spike whole blood to a concentration of 2.0 μmol/L. 40 μL of blood was spotted out on to filter paper (903, Whatman) and allowed to dry at ambient temperature. Stock internal standard solution containing 20 μmol/L of [^{2}H$_9$]-isovalerylcarnitine was prepared in 30% acetonitrile and diluted 1 in 10 to prepare a working internal standard solution.

We tested 122 newborn screening spots from healthy controls and 33 newborn screening samples with C5 results above the analytical cut-off value. During the pilot study the cut-off value was 1.0 μmol/L and this was increased to 2.0 μmol/L following review of the evidence. Confirmatory investigations were performed on all presumptive positive samples and included urinary organic acid analysis, derivatised blood spot acylcarnitines and DNA analysis for the benign mutation. All blood spot samples were collected between days 5 and 8 of age. Blood taken from a heel prick is spotted on to filter paper and transported to the screening laboratory via courier or first class post. Blood spot samples were stored at room temperature until analysis.

A 3.2 mm filter paper disc containing approximately 3.1 μL of whole blood was punched from each dried blood spot into a 96-well polypropylene plate. Samples were extracted for 20 min with 150 μL of 30% acetonitrile containing 2.0 μmol/L [^{2}H$_9$]-isovalerylcarnitine internal standard.

The hardware configuration includes a Waters Premier XE triple quadrupole mass spectrometer equipped with ESI source operating in positive ion mode at a capillary voltage of 3,500. The source temperature was 120 °C, desolvation gas temperature 350 °C and gas flow 800 L/h. Optimised cone voltage was 35 and collision energy 21. All data was acquired in multiple reaction monitoring mode (MRM) with a dwell time of 20 ms per channel. The transitions monitored were 246 > 85 and 255 > 85.

Chromatography was performed on a Waters Acquity UPLC. Isovalerylcarnitine, pivaloylcarnitine, valerylcarnitine and 2-methylbutyrylcarnitine were separated isocrati-

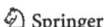

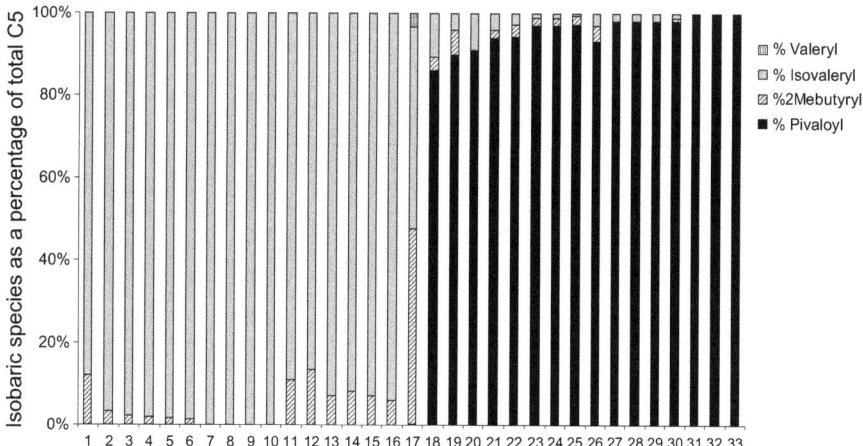

Fig. 1 Isobaric species as a percentage of total C5 in 33 presumptive positive blood spot samples. Samples 1–10 are TP's, samples 11–17 are FP's and samples 18–33 are FP due to pivaloylcarnitine (one FP sample was not available for analysis)

cally by injecting sample extract (10 μL) onto an Acquity BEC C18 column (1.7 μm, 2.1 × 100 mm) fitted with a Vanguard BEH C18 pre-column (1.8 μm, 2.1 × 5.0 mm). The column assembly was maintained at 40 °C. Mobile phase was composed of 0.1% tridecafluoroheptanoic acid (74%) and 0.1% tridecafluoroheptanoic acid in acetontrile (26%) and the flow rate was 450 μL/min. The total run time was 8.0 min and inject-to-inject time was 9.0 min. Isovalerylcarnitine, pivaloylcarnitine, valerylcarnitine and 2-methylbutyrylcarnitine eluted with retention times of 4.0, 4.2, 4.6 and 5.0 min, respectively.

Figure 1 shows the 2 μmol/L blood spot standard and two patients with presumptive positive results for IVA, a FP due to the presence of pivaloylcarnitine and a TP with increased isovalerylcarnitine.

Results

Ion suppression experiments demonstrated that in blood spots the main region of ion suppression occurred between 6.0 and 6.2 min, with no significant ion suppression occurring near the compounds of interest. The assay was linear to at least 10 μmol/L isovalerylcarnitine, intra- and interassay precision were <6% for all four analytes and carry-over was <0.1%. The limit of detection (mean plus 3SD of blank) and the limit of quantification (mean plus 10SD of blank) were 0.06 and 0.2 μmol/L, respectively. Reference ranges (non-parametric, $n = 122$) were determined for each analyte and as % of total C5 they were 44–80%, 19–54%, <3% and <2% for isovalerylcarnitine, 2-methylbutyrylcarnitine, valerylcarnitine and pivaloylcarnitine, respectively.

To assess whether second tier testing would be effective, we analysed the C5 isobars in 33 of the 34 presumptive positive samples identified by the English Newborn Blood Spot Screening (NBSS) program between 2012 and 2016 (one FP sample was not available for analysis). Of these samples, 18 were identified during the pilot study when the cut-off value was 1.0 μmol/L and 16 were identified post pilot when the cut-off value was 2.0 μmol/L. Confirmatory investigations were performed on all samples and included urinary organic acid analysis, derivatised blood spot acylcarnitines and DNA analysis for the 932C > T (A282V) mutation. Table 1 summarises the outcome data for the 33 presumptive positive samples identified by the English NBSS programme.

Of the 18 presumptive positive samples identified during the pilot using a cut-off value of 1.0 μmol/L, 4 were confirmed as TP's and 14 as FP's. Analysis of C5 isobars on these samples demonstrated that 6/14 FP's contained predominantly pivaloylcarnitine (mean 94%, median 96%, range 86–98%). The inclusion of C5 isobar analysis as a second tier test would have increased the PPV from 22.2 to 33.3%. In the post pilot study, using a cut-off value of 2.0 μmol/L, 6 were confirmed as TP's and 10 as FP's. Analysis of C5 isobars on these samples demonstrated that 10/10 contained predominantly pivaloylcarnitine (mean 97%, median 98%, range 90–100%). The inclusion of C5 isobar analysis as a second tier test would have increased the PPV from 38 to 100%. Figure 1 shows the isobaric species as a percentage of total C5 in 33 of the presumptive positive blood spot samples (one sample was not available for analysis) and demonstrates the ability of the test to discriminate between the TP cases of IVA, and the FP's due to pivaloylcarnitine. Samples 1–10 are TP's, samples 11–17 are FP's and samples 18–33 are FP's due to pivaloylcarnitine.

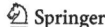

Table 1 Summary of results from 34 newborn blood spot screening samples with presumptive positive result for Isovaleric Acidaemia

Case	Initial C5 on screen µmol/L	% of total C5 isobars				Mutation analysis	Diagnostic C5	Urine organic acids	Additional information	Outcome
		Pivaloyl	Methylbutyryl	Isovaleryl	Valeryl					
1	1.4	98	4	3	0	c.941C>T not detected	NAD	Not measured		FP
2	1.3	0	6	94	0	c.941C>T not detected	0.15 (<0.3)	Trace IVG		FP
3	1.0	0	7	93	0	c.941C>T not detected	0.24 (<0.3)	Trace IVG		FP
4	2.0	0	47	49	3	Not tested	1.42 (<1.2)	NAD		FP
5	1.5	94	2	4	0	c.941C>T not detected	1.54 (<1.2)	NAD		FP
6	1.3	94	3	3	0	c.941C>T not detected	1.54 (<1.2)	NAD		FP
7	1.1	86	3	11	0	c.941C>T not detected	2.3 (<1.2)	NAD		FP
8	1.1	0	13	87	0	c.941C>T not detected	0.45 (<0.5)	1.2 (<2.6)		FP
9	1.0	0	7	93	0	c.941C>T not detected	0.46 (<0.5)	1.8 (<2.6)		FP
10	1.3	0	8	92	0	c.941C>T not detected	0.49 (<0.5)	0.7 (<2.6)		FP
11	1.2	0	11	89	0	c.941C>T not detected	0.17 (<0.5)	0.5 (<2.6)	Breastfed	FP
12	1.9	97	2	1	0	c.941C>T not detected	0.79 (<0.6)	0.4 (<2.6)	Maternal pivampicillin	FP
13	3.6	97	2	1	0	c.941C>T not detected	0.96	0.3 (<2.6)	Maternal pivampicillin	FP
14	1.3					c.941C>T not detected	Not detected	1.1 (<2.6)	No sample for analysis of isobars. SBCAD deficiency	FP
15	11.9	0	0	100	0	c.941C>T not detected	8.4 (<0.3)	Increased IVG		TP
16	1.1	0	2	98	0	c.941C>T not detected	1.6 (<0.5)	54.6 (<2.6)	No antibiotics. Breastfed + formula	TP
17	1.4	0	3	97	0	c.941C>T not detected	2.0 (<0.5)	4.9 (<2.6)		TP
18	6.7	0	12	88	0	Heterozygous for c.941C>T	7.4 (<0.3)	82.3 (<2.6)		TP
19	64.0	0	0	100	0	Homozygous for c.280G>A	13.3 (<0.5)	Not analysed	Sibling of known patient. Diagnosed pre NBS	TP
20	70.0	0	0	100	0	Homozygous for c.367G>A homozygous	8.9 (<0.5)	Increased IVG	Sibling of known patient. Diagnosed pre NBS	TP
21	2.9	0	2	98	0	Homozygous for c.941C>T	5.9 (<0.5)	Increased IVG		TP
22	28.4	0	0	100	0	Known family	13.9 (<0.5)	Increased IVG	Sibling of known patient	TP
23	3.9	0	1	99	0	Heterozygous for c.941C>T	2.6 (<0.5)	Increased IVG	Breastfed	TP
24	1.1	0	2	98	0	c.941C>T not detected	3.7 (<0.5)	Increased IVG	Sibling of known patient	TP
25	2.1	90	6	4	0	c.941C>T not detected	0.6 (<0.5)	NAD		FP
26	1.9	97	2	1	0	Not done	1.5 (<0.5)	NAD	Maternal antibiotics	FP
27	2.3	98	0	2	0	c.941C>T not detected	0.3 (<0.5)	NAD		FP
28	2.3	98	0	2	0	c.941C>T not detected	0.13 (<0.5)	NAD	Breastfed. Mum using Mustela cream	FP
29	3.0	98	0	2	0	c.941C>T not detected	1.4 (<0.3)	NAD		FP
30	4.1	98	1	1	0	c.941C>T not detected	NAD	NAD	Lanolin nipple cream	FP
31	4.4	100	0	0	0	c.941C>T not detected	0.84 (<0.5)	NAD	Maternal antibiotics	FP
32	5.4	100	0	0	0	c.941C>T not detected	1.11 (<0.5)	NAD		FP
33	5.8	100	0	0	0	c.941C>T not detected	0.56 (<0.5)	NAD		FP
34	2.1	2	91	0	9	c.941C>T not detected	1.08 (<0.3)	NAD	Maternal pivmecillinam	FP

Key: Bold = samples collected during pilot

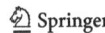

Discussion

The impact of FP screening results has been considered previously. One recent study conducted by health economists reported that whilst patients would wish to avoid the possibility of a FP result if they could, it was not considered to be a major factor. Conversely a study that looked at the outcome of actual FP cases determined an increased parental stress index score, a significant and lasting increase in parental anxiety and an increase in hospital stays of the screen positive children (21% versus 10%) (Bonham 2013). It is evident that screening has the potential to do harm as well as good and so it is important to develop strategies to minimise FP results as well as FN's.

Although the mean concentration of isovalerylcarnitine in the 10 TP samples was 19.1 μmol/L, the median concentration was only 5.3 μmol/L and the range 1.1–70 μmol/L. In comparison, the FP results due to pivaloylcarnitine had a mean initial C5 result of 2.4 μmol/L, median of 2.1 μmol/L and range 1.4–4.4 μmol/L. Data from 173 screening laboratories registered with the CLIR Region 4 website (https://www.clir-r4s.org/) indicates that the 99th centile of C5 in the normal population is 0.38 μmol/L, whilst the 5th centile of the IVA disease range is 0.48 μmol/L. Based on this data CLIR suggests a target range of 0.38–0.48 μmol/L for the C5 cut-off value which is approximately 4.5 times lower than that used in England.

The incidence of FP results due to pivaloylcarnitine is likely to be directly influenced by the prescribing patterns of common pivaloyl containing drugs, such as Pivmecillinam, which is used to treat bacterial infections such as lower tract urinary infections. In July 2012, GP practices in England wrote 2,408 prescriptions for Pivmecillinam whereas in July 2016 this had increased almost fivefold to 11,045. If use of this drug continues to grow at the current rate, the frequency with which FP results due to pivaloylcarnitine occur is also likely to increase. Recent guidance published by Public Health England (2016) recommending pivmecillinam as an alternative therapy when widespread bacterial resistance to ampicillin, amoxicillin and trimethoprim is reported, supports the likelihood of this. Prescribing patterns also vary geographically, with many CCGs in the south of England currently not prescribing the drug at all, compared with relatively frequent use by Airedale, Wharfedale and Craven, Greater Preston and Chorley and South Ribble CCGs (107, 88, 88 and 87 per 1,000 items of Penicillin) (Powell-Smith and Goldacre 2015). This could lead to small clusters of FP results in certain regions and indeed the 8 FP results identified post pilot have originated from the following screening laboratories: Yorkshire ($n = 1$), Sheffield ($n = 4$), Manchester ($n = 2$), West Midlands ($n = 1$), Bristol ($n = 1$) and South East Thames ($n = 1$). Whilst the latter case had no history of antibiotic use (mum was found to be using Mustela nursing balm which contains pivalic acid), at least five of the other cases were confirmed as being linked to maternal antibiotic use. Evidence indicates that the use of pivmecillinam is likely to increase throughout the rest of Europe too: it is now recommended as the treatment for uncomplicated UTIs by the Infectious Diseases Society of America, the European Society for Clinical Microbiology and Infectious Diseases and the European Association of Urology (Dewar et al. 2014).

It can be difficult to draw firm conclusions when only limited numbers of true cases are available. The data collected on samples post pilot, with a cut-off value of 2.0 μmol/L, indicate that incorporation of C5 isobars as second tier test would increase the PPV to 100%. However, it is important to remember that during this time approximately 1 million babies have been screened and 16 screen positive samples identified, 10 of which were FP due to pivaloylcarnitine.

The methodology described here can reliably identify FP IVA screening results due to the presence of pivaloylcarnitine. It is a simple, rapid and robust method that could easily be implemented by newborn screening laboratories. In our opinion, the inclusion of this method as a second tier screening test for IVA will significantly reduce the number of FP results and prevent unnecessary stress and anxiety to parents. In addition, the cost of implementing this second tier test is marginal in comparison to the expense associated with an unnecessary clinical referral.

Synopsis

Introduction of C5 isobars as a second tier screening test for Isovaleric Acidaemia has the potential to significantly reduce the FP rate.

General Rules

The name of the corresponding author: Rachel Carling.
A competing interest statement: No competing interests.
Details of funding N/A.

Conflict of Interest

Rachel Carling, Deborah Burden, Ian Hutton, Rachel Randle, Kate John and Jim Bonham declare no conflict of interest.

This article does not contain any studies with human or animal subjects performed by any of the authors.

All procedures followed were in accordance with the ethical standards of the responsible committee on human experimentation (institutional and national) and with the

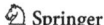

Helsinki Declaration of 1975, as revised in 2000 (5). Informed consent was obtained from all patients for being included in the study.

Details of the contributions of individual authors:

Rachel Carling performed the data analysis, researched the literature and wrote the first draft of the manuscript. All authors contributed to the data interpretation, review and approval of the manuscript.

References

Abdenur JE, Chamoles NA, Guinle AE et al (1998) False positive result due to pivaloylcarnitine in a newborn screening programme. J Inherit Metab Dis 21:624–630

Boemer F, Schoos R, de Halleux V et al (2014) Surprising causes of C5-carnitine false positive results in newborn screening. Mol Gen Metab 111:52–54

Bonham JR (2013) Impact of new screening technologies: should we screen and does phenotype influence this decision? J Inherit Metab Dis 36:681–686

Dewar S, Reed L, Koerner R (2014) Emerging clinical role of pivmecillinam in the treatment of urinary tract infection in the context of multidrug-resistant bacteria. J Antimicrob Chemother 69(2):303–308

Ensenauer R, Vockley J, Willard JM et al (2004) A common mutation is associated with a mild, potentially asymptomatic phenotype in patients with isovaleric acidemia diagnosed by newborn screening. Am J Hum Genet 75:1136–1142

Moorthie S, Cameron L, Sagoo G, Burton H (2013) Birth prevalence of five inherited metabolic diseases. A systematic review. PHG Foundation

Powell-Smith A, Goldacre B (2015) OpenPrescribing.Net

Public Health England (2016) Management of infection guidance for primary care for consultation and local adaptation

Tanaka K (1990) Isovaleric academia: personal history, clinical survey and study of molecular basis. Prog Clin Biol Res 321:273–290

Vockley J, Parimoo B, Nagao M, Tanaka K (1992) Identification of the molecular defects responsible for the various genotypes of isovaleric acidemia. Prog Clin Biol Res 375:533–540

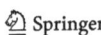

JIMD Reports
DOI 10.1007/8904_2017_29

Open-Label Single-Sequence Crossover Study Evaluating Pharmacokinetics, Efficacy, and Safety of Once-Daily Dosing of Nitisinone in Patients with Hereditary Tyrosinemia Type 1

Nathalie Guffon · Anders Bröijersén ·
Ingrid Palmgren · Mattias Rudebeck · Birgitta Olsson

Received: 26 January 2017 / Revised: 12 April 2017 / Accepted: 18 April 2017 / Published online: 23 June 2017
© The Author(s) 2017

Abstract *Background*: Although nitisinone is successfully used to treat hereditary tyrosinemia type 1 (HT-1) with the recommended twice-daily dosing, data describing a long half-life motivate less frequent dosing. Therefore, in agreement with the Pharmacovigilance Risk Assessment Committee at the European Medicines Agency, this study was performed to investigate the switch to once-daily dosing.

Methods: This open-label, non-randomized, single-sequence crossover study evaluated the pharmacokinetics, efficacy, and safety of once-daily compared to twice-daily dosing of nitisinone in patients with HT-1 (NCT02323529). Well-controlled patients of <2, 2 to <12, 12 to <18, and ≥18 years of age who were on twice-daily dosing were eligible for participation. Nitisinone and succinylacetone levels were determined from dry blood spots by tandem mass spectrometry. The primary endpoint was C_{min} of nitisinone after ≥4 weeks of treatment on each dosing regimen. Secondary objectives were evaluation of efficacy and safety during each dosing regimen.

Results: In total, 19 patients were enrolled and 17 included in the per-protocol analysis set. The mean (SD) nitisinone C_{min} decreased by 23%, from 26.4 (10.2) to 21.2 (9.9) μmol/L in dry blood spot samples (not equivalent to plasma concentrations), when patients switched from twice- to once-daily dosing. There was no apparent age- or body-weight-related trend in the degree of C_{min} decrease. No patient had quantifiable succinylacetone levels during the once-daily treatment period, indicating efficacious treatment. All adverse events were mild or moderate and judged unrelated to nitisinone.

Conclusion: The switch to once-daily treatment with nitisinone appeared efficacious and safe in the treatment of patients with HT-1.

Abbreviations

AE	Adverse event
C_{max}	Maximum concentration
C_{min}	Minimum concentration
HT-1	Hereditary tyrosinemia type 1
LLOQ	Lower limit of quantification
SA	Succinylacetone

Introduction

Hereditary tyrosinemia type 1 (HT-1, OMIM reference 276700) is a rare metabolic disorder with an incidence of 1 in 100,000 worldwide (Hutchesson et al. 1996). The disease is caused by mutations in the *FAH* gene causing defects in fumarylacetoacetate hydrolase (FAH, EC 3.7.1.2), the final enzyme of the pathway responsible for degradation of tyrosine. As a consequence, the catabolic toxic intermediates maleylacetoacetate and fumarylacetoacetate accumulate and convert into succinylacetone (SA) and succinylacetoacetate causing liver damage including hepatocellular carcinoma as well as kidney dysfunction, neurological problems, and shorter life expectancy (Lindblad et al. 1977; Mitchell et al. 2001; van Ginkel et al. 2016).

Communicated by: Johannes Häberle

N. Guffon
Centre de Référence des Maladies Héréditaires du Métabolisme,
Hôpital Femme Mère Enfant, 59 Boulevard Pinel,
69677 Bron, France

A. Bröijersén (✉) · I. Palmgren · M. Rudebeck · B. Olsson
Swedish Orphan Biovitrum (Sobi), 112 76 Stockholm, Sweden
e-mail: anders.broijersen@sobi.com

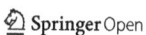

Nitisinone, also known as NTBC (Orfadin®, Sobi), is a reversible inhibitor of 4-hydroxyphenylpyruvate dioxygenase (HPPD, EC 1.13.11.27), an enzyme upstream of FAH in the tyrosine catabolic pathway that prevents accumulation of toxic metabolites (Schulz et al. 1993). To date, nitisinone is the only approved substance for the treatment of HT-1, and in combination with a low-tyrosine diet and special amino acid supplements, the treatment has resulted in a greater than 90% survival rate of patients with HT-1 (Larochelle et al. 2012). The drug is well tolerated with few side effects and the only alternative treatment option is liver transplantation. Early diagnosis is important to allow early treatment initiation and better long-term outcome and is facilitated in many countries by newborn screening, ideally using SA as a disease marker (De Jesus et al. 2014; Mayorandan et al. 2014).

The clinical study upon which the marketing approval of nitisinone was based practiced twice-daily dosing (Holme and Lindstedt 2000), which also appears as the most commonly practiced dosing frequency (Mayorandan et al. 2014). The long half-life in plasma, median 54 h (range: 39–86 h), has however motivated some clinicians to reduce dosing frequency to once-daily (Hall et al. 2001; McKiernan 2013). Moreover, once-daily dosing is advised in recent recommendations (de Laet et al. 2013), but the suitability of switching from twice- to once-daily dosing has not been properly documented; there is, however, one small study including nine patients reporting that once-daily dosing may be as effective as a multiple-dose regimen (Schlune et al. 2012). It was therefore agreed with the Pharmacovigilance Risk Assessment Committee (PRAC) at the European Medicines Agency (EMA) to perform the study presented here, with the purpose of investigating the effect on nitisinone serum concentrations and clinical outcome, when switching patients of all ages with HT-1 to the less frequent once-daily dosing regimen, which may be preferable from a convenience and compliance perspective (Iskedjian et al. 2002; Coleman et al. 2012).

Subjects and Methodology

Subjects

Patients eligible for the study were male or female patients of all ages diagnosed with HT-1 who were well controlled on twice-daily, or more frequent, nitisinone dosing according to the investigator, and who had stable laboratory values: alkaline phosphatase, alanine aminotransferase, aspartate aminotransferase, bilirubin, and international normalized ratio. Women of childbearing age were to use contraception to allow study inclusion. Individuals with

prior periods of once-daily dosing were excluded due to the risk of selection bias. Additional reasons for exclusion were: participation in any other interventional clinical study within 3 months prior to inclusion in this study, pregnancy, breast feeding, previous liver transplant, or patients who within the past 4 weeks prior to inclusion started any new medication for a previously undiagnosed illness, any foreseeable inability to cooperate with given instructions or study procedures, or any medical condition that in the opinion of the investigator made the patient unsuitable for inclusion. The first patient was included in December 2014 and the last patient's last visit was in September 2015.

The study (www.clinicaltrials.gov identifier: NCT02323529) was conducted according to International Conference on Harmonisation-Good Clinical Practice guidelines and the Declaration of Helsinki and was approved by relevant regulatory authorities and independent ethics committees. Informed consent was obtained from the patient or patient's legal representative (for patients under the age of 18) prior to any study intervention.

Study Design

This was an open-label, non-randomized, single-sequence crossover study aiming to enroll a minimum of 20 patients with preferably 5 patients, but minimum 3 patients, in each age group (infants: <2 years of age, children: 2 years to <12 years of age, adolescents: 12 years to <18 years of age, adults: ≥18 years of age). Patients were enrolled from six sites in Belgium, Denmark, France, Germany, and Sweden. The study was divided into three periods: screening, treatment period 1, and treatment period 2 (Fig. 1a). At screening, if SA was quantifiable in urine or serum samples taken locally or in case of other signs of inadequate dosing, the patient's nitisinone dose was to be adjusted and screening was repeated (maximum one time). Otherwise, the patient started treatment period 1 during which nitisinone was dosed twice-daily for at least 4 weeks. If SA was quantifiable at the end of treatment period 1, an adjusted higher dose was used for an additional 4 weeks, and if the SA levels were still quantifiable by the end of this period the patient was to be withdrawn from the study. Patients with no quantifiable SA, or no other signs of inadequate dosing, at the end of treatment period 1 continued to treatment period 2, during which nitisinone was dosed once-daily for at least 4 weeks.

Study Intervention and Pharmacokinetic Assessment

Capsules of 2, 5, or 10 mg nitisinone were provided for the study. The individual nitisinone dose was the one pre-

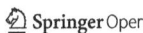

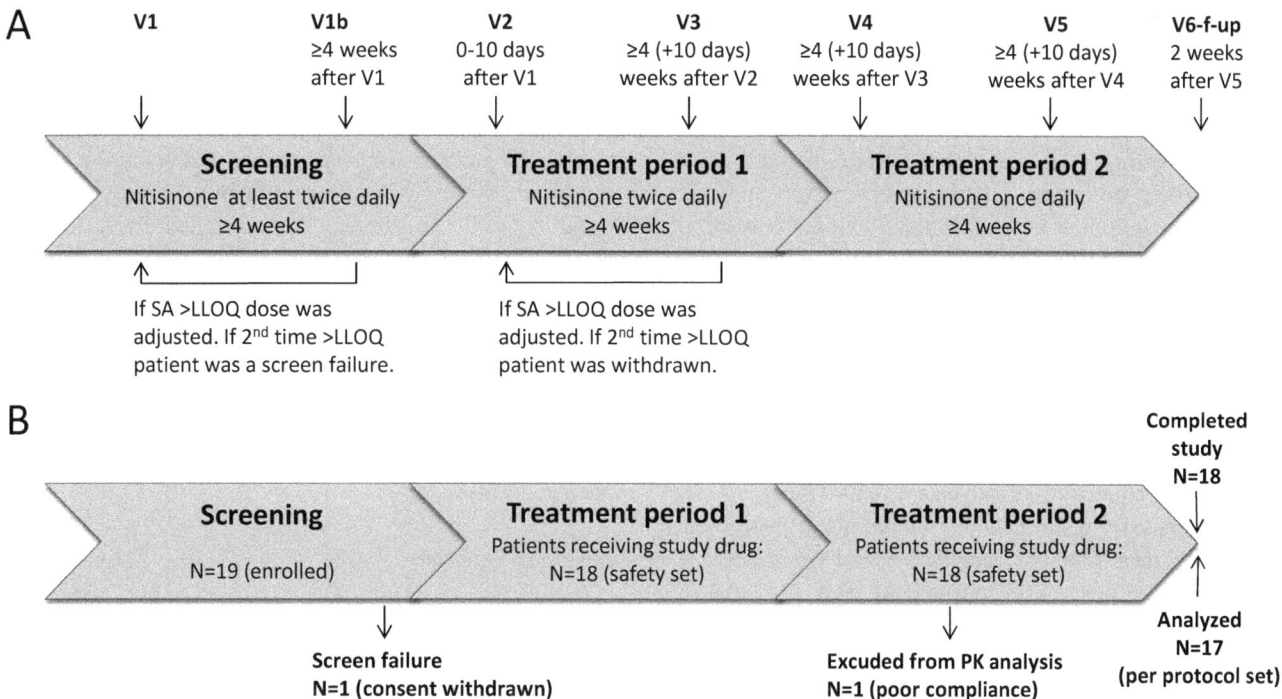

Fig. 1 Study design and patient disposition. (a) Study design. (b) Patient disposition during the study

scribed by the treating physician during the screening period. The mode of administration (swallowing the capsules whole or mixing the contents with food or drinks) matched each patients' prior habits and was noted in the case report form. Once patients entered treatment period 2 (once-daily dosing), the dose was taken in the morning. Considering the involvement of pediatric patients, blood sampling (volumes and occasions) was kept to a minimum and only C_{min} (minimum concentration) and C_{max} (maximum concentration) were studied, as these were the only two variables affected by a change in dosing frequency. Thus no full PK evaluation was performed. C_{min} was determined in samples taken immediately before dosing and because determination of C_{max} would have required blood sampling over several hours, a near maximum concentration was determined from a sample taken in the interval between 3 and 4 h after dosing. The choice of this sampling time was based on data from the only study with PK data for nitisinone at steady-state. That study, however, used a liquid formulation of nitisinone (Olsson et al. 2015). Samples for both C_{min} and C_{max} were taken at the end of each treatment period, i.e., at visits 3 and 5 (Fig. 1a).

Outcome Measures

The primary study objective was to evaluate the steady-state exposure to nitisinone during once- and twice-daily dosing by assessing the C_{min} after at least 4 weeks of treatment on each dosing regimen, defined as the concen-

tration in the dry blood spot (DBS) sample taken immediately before dosing. Secondary endpoints related to the primary objective were assessment of C_{max} of nitisinone and the C_{max}/C_{min} ratio after at least 4 weeks of treatment on each dosage regimen. Additional secondary objectives were to evaluate the efficacy of nitisinone during once-daily dosing by assessing concentrations of SA after at least 4 weeks of treatment and nitisinone levels and C_{min} if SA was above the lower limit of quantification (LLOQ). An analytical method for the determination of nitisinone and SA in DBS, using liquid extraction followed by mass spectrometry (LC-MS/MS), was validated over concentration ranges of 0.500–120 μmol/L (nitisinone) and 0.250–50.0 μmol/L (SA). The limit of quantification in our assay was 0.250 μmol/L SA which was considered sufficiently low with regard to normal DBS SA levels measuring up to 1 μmol/L or more (Allard et al. 2004; la Marca et al. 2008; Turgeon et al. 2008; Dhillon et al. 2011; Yang et al. 2017). Central laboratory measurement of nitisinone and SA levels were made in the DBSs from visits 1 (only SA), 3, and 5. A conversion of whole blood (DBS) concentrations to serum concentrations, taking individual hematocrit values into account, was originally planned for both nitisinone and SA. This was, however, not performed because factors other than hematocrit values could influence these results and the method was not validated to allow such conversion. Moreover, for SA a conversion was not applicable since all concentrations in the DBS samples were below the LLOQ. For nitisinone, the

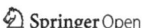

actual serum concentration can be estimated to be approximately 1.6 times higher than the DBS concentrations (Sander et al. 2011).

In addition to the DBS samples that were sent to a central laboratory at the end of the study, blood (serum/plasma/DBS) or urine samples were tested in local laboratories according to local routine with the purpose of evaluating whether dose adjustments were necessary during the course of the study.

Safety Assessments

Evaluation of safety during once- and twice-daily dosing was also included as a secondary objective. This was assessed by collection of adverse events (AEs), routine clinical chemistry tests including serum alpha fetoprotein, hepatic and renal function, coagulation, and serum tyrosine. All enrolled patients who received at least one dose of study drug were included in the safety analysis set. AEs were collected until the last visit whether or not the event was considered to be treatment related and serious adverse events (SAEs) were collected until 28 days past the last dose.

Statistics

Due to the low prevalence of HT-1, the sample size was based on feasibility rather than on statistical power considerations. A minimum enrollment of 20 patients was planned.

All data were summarized descriptively. In addition, for the PK data, the geometric mean, associated 95% CI (confidence interval) for C_{min} and C_{max} and the C_{max}/C_{min} ratio were calculated. Statistical analyses were performed using SAS software Version 9.1 or later (SAS Institute, Inc. Cary, North Carolina, USA).

Results

Demographics and Baseline Characteristics

In total, 19 patients were enrolled in the study. However, one patient withdrew her consent before entering treatment period 1, and one patient was excluded from the PK analysis due to poor compliance in the once-daily period, leaving 18 patients in the safety-set and 17 patients in the per-protocol set (Fig. 1b). The mean (SD) age was 13.2 (7.1) years, and ranged from 1.3 to 24.0 years. Due to recruitment difficulties, only two patients were included in the youngest age group while five to six patients were included in the other age groups. The gender distribution was equal (Table 1).

Nitisinone Exposure

The nitisinone steady-state exposure during once- and twice-daily dosing was estimated by assessing the C_{min} and C_{max} values. The mean (SD) nitisinone C_{min} was lower (21.2 [9.9] μmol/L) for the once-daily treatment period compared to the twice-daily treatment period (26.4 [10.2] μmol/L) (Fig. 2a). All age groups showed a similar trend of lower C_{min} during once-daily compared to twice-daily dosing (not shown). The geometric mean treatment ratio (C_{min} once daily/C_{min} twice daily) was 0.77 (95% CI: 0.68, 0.87), corresponding to a 23% decrease in C_{min} after switching from twice- to once-daily dosing. Note that these concentrations assessed from DBS samples should not be directly compared to the serum concentrations mentioned in the treatment recommendations (de Laet et al. 2013).

The mean (SD) C_{max} was similar for the twice- (31.1 [14.3] μmol/L) and once-daily (29.3 [11.6] μmol/L) treatment period. However, it should be noted that the exact C_{max} was not determined in this study. For drugs like

Table 1 Demographics and baseline characteristics (safety set)

	<2 years ($N = 2$)	2 to <12 years ($N = 5$)	12 to <18 years ($N = 5$)	≥18 years ($N = 6$)	All ($N = 18$)
Age (years)					
Mean (SD)	1.5 (0.2)	7.7 (2.4)	13.9 (1.2)	21.1 (2.3)	13.2 (7.1)
Min, max	1.3, 1.6	5.0, 11.0	13.0, 15.4	19.0, 24.0	1.3, 24.0
Sex					
Male	2 (100.0%)	4 (80.0%)	2 (40.0%)	1 (16.7%)	9 (50.0%)
Female	0	1 (20.0%)	3 (60.0%)	5 (83.3%)	9 (50.0%)
Age at HT-1 diagnosis (months)					
Mean (SD)	8.0 (2.1)	8.2 (6.4)	7.0 (4.1)	8.8 (5.3)	8.1 (4.8)
Age at nitisinone treatment start (months)					
Mean (SD)	8.5 (2.1)	8.2 (6.4)	7.2 (4.3)	15.3 (14.3)	10.3 (9.4)

SD standard deviation

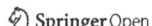

nitisinone with a linear relationship between dose and plasma concentration (linear pharmacokinetics) a change in dosing frequency with maintained total dose does not change the overall average drug concentration in the dosage interval but rather the fluctuations around the average. Once-daily dosing was therefore expected to result in an increase in C_{max} of the same magnitude as the decrease in C_{min} compared to twice-daily dosing. For this reason these results indicate that for many patients the optimum sampling time for determination of C_{max} was not within 3–4 h after dosing, since in general no such increase was observed.

The once-daily/twice-daily C_{min} ratios varied among patients and plotting the data by age, instead of body-weight, provided overall similar results (Fig. 2b and not shown). Due to the low number of patients and the fact that some patients with higher weight (also older) had similar ratios as the patient with the lowest weight (youngest), it can be concluded that the once-daily/twice-daily C_{min} ratios appeared to be independent of patient weight and age.

No patient required a dose adjustment after switching to once daily dosing. Thus, the mean (SD) prescribed daily nitisinone dose was the same, 0.78 (0.27) mg/kg ($N = 18$), for both the twice-daily and the once-daily dosing periods (not shown).

Efficacy of Nitisinone Treatment

Since quantifiable levels of SA indicate insufficient inhibition of HPPD, treatment efficacy was determined by the proportion of patients with quantifiable serum or urine SA levels as assessed by both local and central laboratory, after at least 4 weeks of once-daily nitisinone treatment. No patient had SA levels above the LLOQ at the end of the once-daily treatment period. However, in a local plasma

sample at the end of the twice-daily treatment period, one patient had SA levels above LLOQ. After 4 weeks on an increased dose, and no detectable SA, the patient entered the once-daily period.

Safety

Overall, 15 patients (83.3%) experienced at least 1 AE during the study (Table 2). Thirteen patients (72.2%) experienced at least 1 AE during the twice-daily treatment period and 11 patients (61.1%) experienced at least 1 AE during the once-daily treatment period. All AEs were mild or moderate in intensity. One patient experienced an SAE (gastroenteritis) during the twice-daily treatment period. No AE (including the SAE) was considered by the investigator to be related to the nitisinone treatment. No patient had any clinically significant change in any laboratory parameter, including serum tyrosine levels, or an AE associated with a safety laboratory parameter.

Most AEs were within the system organ class "infections and infestations"; 8 patients with 8 events in the twice-daily treatment period and 5 patients with 5 events in the once-daily treatment period. In conclusion there were no apparent differences in either the number or the type of AEs between twice- and once-daily dosing periods.

Discussion

In this prospective single-sequence crossover study on 18 patients with HT-1 that compared the efficacy, safety, and steady-state exposure of nitisinone during once- and twice-daily dosing, once-daily treatment appeared as efficacious and safe as twice-daily treatment. There were no clinically

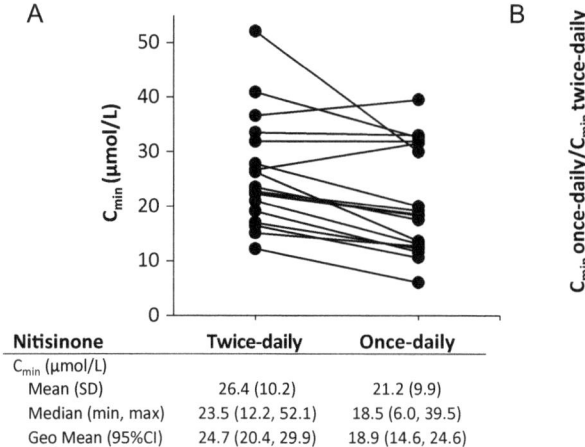

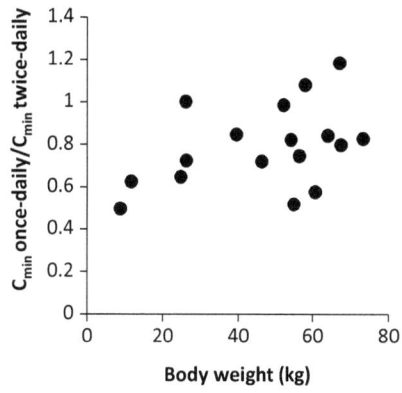

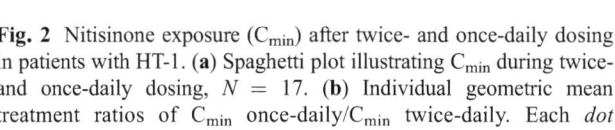

Nitisinone	Twice-daily	Once-daily
C_{min} (μmol/L)		
Mean (SD)	26.4 (10.2)	21.2 (9.9)
Median (min, max)	23.5 (12.2, 52.1)	18.5 (6.0, 39.5)
Geo Mean (95%CI)	24.7 (20.4, 29.9)	18.9 (14.6, 24.6)

Fig. 2 Nitisinone exposure (C_{min}) after twice- and once-daily dosing in patients with HT-1. (**a**) Spaghetti plot illustrating C_{min} during twice- and once-daily dosing, $N = 17$. (**b**) Individual geometric mean treatment ratios of C_{min} once-daily/C_{min} twice-daily. Each *dot* represents one patient, $N = 17$. *CI* confidence interval, C_{min} minimum concentration, defined as pre-dose concentration, *CV* coefficient of variation, *SD* standard deviation

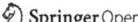

Table 2 Number of adverse events (AEs) (safety set)

Category	Twice-daily treatment period ($N = 18$)	Once-daily treatment period ($N = 18$)	Any treatment period ($N = 18$)
Patients who had an AE	13 (72.2%)	11 (61.1%)	15 (83.3%)
Number of AEs	18	18	36
Patient who had a mild AE	12 (66.7%)	11 (61.1%)	14 (77.8%)
Number of mild AEs	15	16	31
Patients who had a moderate AE	2 (11.1%)	2 (11.1%)	4 (22.2%)
Number of moderate AEs	3	2	5
Patients who had a severe AE	0	0	0
Patients who had a treatment-related AE[a]	0	0	0
Patients who had an SAE	1 (5.6%)	0	1 (5.6%)
Number of SAEs	1	0	1
Patients who had an AE resulting in death	0	0	0

Note: Only AEs after first dose of study drug included. Percentages based on the number of patients in each treatment period

AE adverse event, *SAE* serious adverse event

[a] Relationship judged by the investigator

significant differences in the number or type of AEs between the treatment regimens.

To our knowledge there are no clinical studies to date investigating the optimal dosing frequency of nitisinone in patients with HT-1. Although 1 mg/kg body weight per day divided in two daily doses is presently recommended (Orfadin® summary of product characteristics), once-daily dosing is supported by the long half-life of nitisinone in plasma (median approximately 54 h = 2.3 days) (Hall et al. 2001). A retrospective study on real-life clinical practice in Europe, Turkey, and Israel showed that the dosing frequency varied from once to thrice daily with an average of twice daily (Mayorandan et al. 2014). The availability of PK data in the literature is limited, emphasizing the need of more information in this field. Since the risk of less frequent dosing is a temporary insufficient HPPD blockade with SA breakthrough, C_{min} prior to dosing was chosen as the primary PK endpoint for this study. As expected, according to pharmacokinetic principles, the mean C_{min} measured after once daily dosing was lower than after twice daily dosing. However, there was no breakthrough of SA in this study indicating that once-daily dosing was as efficacious as twice-daily dosing.

In further support of once-daily dosing is a study demonstrating that it was as effective as a multiple-dosing regimen for nine patients with HT-1 (Schlune et al. 2012). Also in favor of once-daily dosing are the preclinical studies showing a slow dissociation rate of the nitisinone-HPPD complex and slow recovery of HPPD enzyme activity, indicating that a temporary decrease in nitisinone serum concentration does not necessarily reflect a propor-tional loss of HPPD inhibition (Ellis et al. 1995; Lock et al. 1996).

A change in dosing frequency with maintained total dose, as in this study, does not change the overall average drug concentration in the dosage interval, only the fluctuations of drug concentration within the interval. The decrease in C_{min} is expected to be mirrored by a corresponding increase in C_{max}. Correct C_{max} determination requires blood sampling over several hours, which was not considered ethical in this study due to the predominantly pediatric population. Therefore, the time for maximum concentrations (t_{max}) was estimated based on previously published nitisinone steady-state levels (Olsson et al. 2015) and samples were taken 3–4 h after dosing. Unfortunately the average C_{max} was similar after switching from twice- to once-daily dosing, indicating that the timing of C_{max} sampling was suboptimal. It was therefore irrelevant to report actual fluctuations during the dosage interval (C_{max}/C_{min} ratios) even though they were included as secondary endpoints.

For practical as well as ethical reasons considering very young children, this study assessed nitisinone levels from DBS (small volumes of blood and less invasive than serum samples). However, it is important to note that the nitisinone levels reported here were, due to practical constraints, not converted to corresponding serum levels as initially planned. For this reason any direct comparison to the recommended serum levels in the treatment of HT-1 would be incorrect. General awareness should be brought to the complexity of converting concentrations in DBS samples to plasma or serum concentrations since the correct

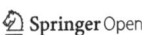

conversion factor needs to be determined for each DBS method at the local laboratory if it is going to be used in therapeutic monitoring.

The low incidence of HT-1 and the fact that most patients are still pediatric pose challenges to the recruitment into clinical studies in this patient population and is a reason for the relatively low number of patients in this study, especially in the younger ages. Despite an extended enrollment period and inquiries for additional patients across Europe to fill the quota in the youngest age group (<2 years of age), no additional patients were found and it was decided to terminate the study with only two infants. The recruitment difficulty can be explained by the fact that this age group covered only 2 years while other age groups had a much wider age span. Moreover during the 2 years the infants also had to be diagnosed and have an established nitisinone treatment ongoing for several months before inclusion, leaving a very short window of recruitment opportunities for infants. Furthermore, after establishing initial treatment, parents might be hesitant to change regimen in these very young children. Thus, a total of 19 patients were enrolled in the study, not 20 as originally planned in the study protocol.

In conclusion, the results of this study contribute to the overall understanding of the flexibility of nitisinone dosing for patients with HT-1. Switching from twice-daily to once-daily dosing proved both safe and efficacious for all patients in this study and is therefore recommended. However, we cannot exclude that some individuals may benefit from more frequent dosing and a switch to once-daily dosing should ideally be carefully monitored.

Acknowledgments First of all we thank the patients who participated in this study and their families. We also thank the principal investigators Dr. Corinne de Laet (Hôpital Universitaire des Enfants Reine Fabiola, Brussels, Belgium), Dr. Clemens Kamrath (Universitätsklinikum Gießen und Marburg, Gießen, Germany), Dr. Allan Lund (Copenhagen University Hospital, Copenhagen, Denmark), Dr. Annika Reims (Queen Silvia Children Hospital, Gothenburg, Sweden), Prof Peter Freisinger (Kreiskliniken Reutlingen, Germany), the lead study coordinator at Kreiskliniken Reutlingen Dinah Lier (Germany), and the study teams at all participating sites. In addition, we thank the study team at Sobi for their contribution to the study and the medical writer, Kristina Lindsten (Sobi), for the assistance with drafting the manuscript.

Disclosures

Nathalie Guffon: Coordinating investigator for the study. NG participated in several clinical trials and have institution contracts including investigators fees from Genzyme Sanofi, Shire HGT, BioMarin, and Sobi.

Anders Bröijersén: Employee of Sobi and holder of Sobi shares.

Ingrid Palmgren: Employee of Sobi and holder of Sobi shares.

Mattias Rudebeck: Employee of Sobi and holder of Sobi shares.

Birgitta Olsson: Employee of Sobi and holder of Sobi shares.

This study was fully funded by Sobi (Swedish Orphan Biovitrum AB [publ]).

Informed Consent

All procedures followed were in accordance with the ethical standards of the responsible committee on human experimentation (institutional and national) and with the Helsinki Declaration of 1975, as revised in 2000 (5). Informed consent was obtained from all patients before being included in the study.

Individual Author Contribution

Nathalie Guffon was the coordinating investigator of the study and substantially contributed to the acquisition and interpretation of data. Nathalie Guffon also actively participated in drafting the manuscript and approved of the final version to be submitted.

Anders Bröijersén contributed to the concept and design of the study and he also analyzed the study results and had the overall medical responsibility during the study. Anders Bröijersén also participated in drafting the manuscript, approved of the final version to be submitted and is corresponding author.

Ingrid Palmgren contributed to the concept and design of the study and she also analyzed the study results with particular focus on all safety aspects. Ingrid Palmgren also participated in drafting the manuscript and approved of the final version to be submitted.

Mattias Rudebeck contributed to the concept and design of the study and he also analyzed the study results. Mattias Rudebeck also participated in drafting the manuscript and approved of the final version to be submitted.

Birgitta Olsson contributed to the concept and design of the study and she also analyzed the study results with particular focus an all pharmacokinetic aspects. Birgitta Olsson also participated in drafting the manuscript and approved of the final version to be submitted.

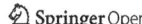

References

Allard P, Grenier A, Korson MS, Zytkovicz TH (2004) Newborn screening for hepatorenal tyrosinemia by tandem mass spectrometry: analysis of succinylacetone extracted from dried blood spots. Clin Biochem 37:1010–1015

Coleman CI, Limone B, Sobieraj DM et al (2012) Dosing frequency and medication adherence in chronic disease. J Manag Care Pharm 18:527–539

De Jesus VR, Adam BW, Mandel D, Cuthbert CD, Matern D (2014) Succinylacetone as primary marker to detect tyrosinemia type I in newborns and its measurement by newborn screening programs. Mol Genet Metab 113:67–75

de Laet C, Dionisi-Vici C, Leonard JV et al (2013) Recommendations for the management of tyrosinaemia type 1. Orphanet J Rare Dis 8:8

Dhillon KS, Bhandal AS, Aznar CP, Lorey FW, Neogi P (2011) Improved tandem mass spectrometry (MS/MS) derivatized method for the detection of tyrosinemia type I, amino acids and acylcarnitine disorders using a single extraction process. Clin Chim Acta 412:873–879

Ellis MK, Whitfield AC, Gowans LA et al (1995) Inhibition of 4-hydroxyphenylpyruvate dioxygenase by 2-(2-nitro-4-trifluorome-thylbenzoyl)-cyclohexane-1,3-dione and 2-(2-chloro-4-methane-sulfonylbenzoyl)-cyclohexane-1,3-dione. Toxicol Appl Pharmacol 133:12–19

Hall MG, Wilks MF, Provan WM, Eksborg S, Lumholtz B (2001) Pharmacokinetics and pharmacodynamics of NTBC (2-(2-nitro-4-fluoromethylbenzoyl)-1,3-cyclohexanedione) and mesotrione, inhibitors of 4-hydroxyphenyl pyruvate dioxygenase (HPPD) following a single dose to healthy male volunteers. Br J Clin Pharmacol 52:169–177

Holme E, Lindstedt S (2000) Nontransplant treatment of tyrosinemia. Clin Liver Dis 4:805–814

Hutchesson AC, Hall SK, Preece MA, Green A (1996) Screening for tyrosinaemia type I. Arch Dis Child Fetal Neonatal Ed 74: F191–F194

Iskedjian M, Einarson TR, MacKeigan LD et al (2002) Relationship between daily dose frequency and adherence to antihypertensive pharmacotherapy: evidence from a meta-analysis. Clin Ther 24:302–316

la Marca G, Malvagia S, Pasquini E et al (2008) The inclusion of succinylacetone as marker for tyrosinemia type I in expanded newborn screening programs. Rapid Commun Mass Spectrom 22:812–818

Larochelle J, Alvarez F, Bussieres JF et al (2012) Effect of nitisinone (NTBC) treatment on the clinical course of hepatorenal tyrosinemia in Quebec. Mol Genet Metab 107:49–54

Lindblad B, Lindstedt S, Steen G (1977) On the enzymic defects in hereditary tyrosinemia. Proc Natl Acad Sci U S A 74:4641–4645

Lock EA, Gaskin P, Ellis MK et al (1996) Tissue distribution of 2-(2-nitro-4-trifluoromethylbenzoyl)cyclohexane-1-3-dione (NTBC): effect on enzymes involved in tyrosine catabolism and relevance to ocular toxicity in the rat. Toxicol Appl Pharmacol 141:439–447

Mayorandan S, Meyer U, Gokcay G et al (2014) Cross-sectional study of 168 patients with hepatorenal tyrosinaemia and implications for clinical practice. Orphanet J Rare Dis 9:107

McKiernan PJ (2013) Nitisinone for the treatment of hereditary tyrosinemia type I. Expert Opin Orphan Drugs 1:491–497

Mitchell GA, Grompe M, Lambert M, Tanguay RM (2001) Hypertyrosinemia. In: Scriver CR, Beaudet AL, Sly WS, Valle D (eds) The metabolic and molecular basis of inherited disease. McGraw Hill, New York, pp 1777–1805

Olsson B, Cox TF, Psarelli EE et al (2015) Relationship between serum concentrations of nitisinone and its effect on homogentisic acid and tyrosine in patients with alkaptonuria. JIMD Rep 24:21–27

Sander J, Janzen N, Terhardt M et al (2011) Monitoring tyrosinaemia type I: blood spot test for nitisinone (NTBC). Clin Chim Acta 412:134–138

Schlune A, Thimm E, Herebian D, Spiekerkoetter U (2012) Single dose NTBC-treatment of hereditary tyrosinemia type I. J Inherit Metab Dis 35:831–836

Schulz A, Ort O, Beyer P, Kleinig H (1993) SC-0051, a 2-benzoyl-cyclohexane-1,3-dione bleaching herbicide, is a potent inhibitor of the enzyme p-hydroxyphenylpyruvate dioxygenase. FEBS Lett 318:162–166

Turgeon C, Magera MJ, Allard P et al (2008) Combined newborn screening for succinylacetone, amino acids, and acylcarnitines in dried blood spots. Clin Chem 54:657–664

van Ginkel WG, Jahja R, Huijbregts SC et al (2016) Neurocognitive outcome in tyrosinemia type 1 patients compared to healthy controls. Orphanet J Rare Dis 11:87

Yang H, Al-Hertani W, Cyr D et al (2017) Hypersuccinylacetonaemia and normal liver function in maleylacetoacetate isomerase deficiency. J Med Genet 54:241–247

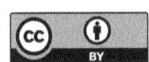
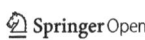

JIMD Reports
DOI 10.1007/8904_2017_34

RESEARCH REPORT

A Rapid Two-Step Iduronate-2-Sulfatatse Enzymatic Activity Assay for MPSII Pharmacokinetic Assessment

Mitra Azadeh · Luying Pan · Yongchang Qiu · Ruben Boado

Received: 6 April 2017 /Revised: 22 May 2017 /Accepted: 30 May 2017 /Published online: 23 June 2017
© SSIEM and Springer-Verlag Berlin Heidelberg 2017

Abstract Clinical studies involving enzyme replacement therapies (ERTs) have increasingly utilized enzymatic activity assays to monitor efficacy and biofunction of the drug; as a result, these assays have become an important part of pharmacokinetic (PK) and pharmacodynamic assessments in ERT trials. This paper presents a two-step enzymatic activity assay for iduronate-2-sulfatase (I2S) (EC 3.1.6.13) which we have optimized to fit in 1 day and to complete in less than 6 h. The rapid assay presented here is a significant improvement over the original two-step method with run time of 24 h which spanned 2 days. The resulting 1 day assay is efficient, robust, reproducible, and better suited for use in pharmacokinetic studies. The method was fully validated in accordance with regulatory agency guidelines so that it could be implemented in PK studies. Validation of the method required additional modifications to circumvent limitations surrounding the calculation of accuracy. This challenge was overcome by developing strategies to determine both the expected and the measured values of validation samples in activity units. Subsequently, the method was validated in accordance with the FDA guidance for the validation of quantitative ligand binding assays (LBAs). Results of method development and optimization with focus on evaluations aimed at reducing the total assay run time as well as a summary of method validation performance are presented in this publication.

Communicated by: Francois Feillet, MD, PhD

M. Azadeh (✉) · L. Pan · Y. Qiu
Shire, 125 Spring Street, Lexington, MA 02421, USA
e-mail: mazadeh@shire.com; lpan@shire.com; yqiu@shire.com

R. Boado
ArmaGen Inc., 26679 Agoura Rd, Calabasas, CA 92302, USA
e-mail: rboado@armagen.com

Introduction

Mucopolysaccharidosis type II (MPSII), or Hunter Syndrome, is a genetically inherited lysosomal storage disease characterized by the deficiency of enzyme I2S. As an X-linked recessive disease, Hunter Syndrome primarily affects males at the approximate rate of 1 out of every 70,000 live births. The deficiency affects the body's ability to break down glycosaminoglycans (GAGs) (Muenzer et al. 2006, 2007), resulting in accumulation of GAGs which causes progressive damage impacting physical appearance, range of motion and mobility, organ function, and in some, cognitive abilities. Recombinant human I2S drugs such as Elaprase (Shire, USA) and Hunterase (Green Cross, South Korea) have been approved as ERTs for the treatment of MPSII. A novel brain penetrating I2S-anti-human insulin receptor IgG fusion compound, AGT-182, which is a chimera of two I2S and one IgG molecules (Lu et al. 2010) is also in evaluation and in a phase I clinical trial (NCT02262338).

Fluorometric enzyme assays have long been employed to measure the activity of I2S as part of pharmaco-dynamic and pharmacokinetic studies of this enzyme (Tolun et al. 2012; Johnson et al. 2013). This paper presents a two-step I2S enzymatic activity assay, modified from a previously published method (Voznyi et al. 2001) which is also fluorometric but differs from most existing assays in a number of ways. The method presented here utilizes 4-methylumbelliferyl α-L-iduronide-2-sulfate (4-MUS) as substrate (Voznyi et al. 2001). 4-MUS has greater specificity towards I2S. Use of 4-MUS is an advantage over other I2S enzymatic assays which utilize 4-methylumbelli-feryl-sulfate (4-MS) (Inoue et al. 1982), a substrate that is hydrolyzed by all sulfatases (Inoue et al. 1982; Hopwood 1979).

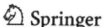

In the first of the two steps, 4-MUS is hydrolyzed by I2S to 4-methylumbelliferyl α-L-iduronide (MUBI). The first step reaction is completely stopped by the phosphate present in the second step reaction buffer (Voznyi et al. 2001), and subsequently in the second step, another lysosomal enzyme, α-L-iduronidase (IDUA) (EC 3.2.1.76), hydrolyzes MUBI to the final product, 4-methylumbelliferone or 4-MU. 4-MU emits fluorescence, and the signal is quantified against a calibration curve prepared with synthetic 4-MU. In a series of evaluations presented in this paper, both reagent concentrations and the incubation times of the two-step assay were optimized to yield a method that is robust, can be performed in only a few hours, costs less, and is hence more suitable for clinical and nonclinical studies.

An earlier version of this assay was validated and used in preclinical studies of AGT-182 in primates (Boado et al. 2014). The primate assay was based on the original method published by Voznyi et al. (2001), without the optimizations presented in this paper. Some of the challenges in the validation of the two-step activity assay for use in regulated studies stemmed from the absence of a typical quantitative calibration curve prepared from the study matrix fortified with the AGT-182. This posed a significant limitation on validating the method since it did not allow for the extrapolation of the validation sample (VS) values in the same units used to spike them. The resulting disparity between the units for the expected versus measured values of VSs (ng/mL or μg/mL versus nmol/h/mL or nmol/h/μg) made it difficult to assess method accuracy. We addressed this limitation by establishing expected values in activity units for each VS which subsequently allowed for the calculation of accuracy as percent recovery of measured versus expected value for each validation parameter. This publication presents optimization strategies used to reformat the assay into a rapid method as well as a summary of method validation performance including accuracy and precision, selectivity, and dilutional linearity.

Materials and Methods

Preparation of Assay Quality Controls

Assay quality controls were prepared at high, medium, and low levels (HQC, MQC, and LQC at 800, 400, and 100 ng/mL, respectively) by adding AGT-182 into a qualified pool of human K₂EDTA plasma. For accuracy and precision runs, VSs were prepared at five levels of upper limit of quantitation (ULOQ, 1,000 ng/mL), HQC, MQC, LQC, and lower limit of quantitation (LLOQ, 50 ng/mL) to span the targeted quantitative range of the assay.

Sample Storage and Preparation

The study plasma samples as well as the assay quality controls were stored at −80 °C. In preparation for the activity assay, plasma samples and the quality controls were thawed on ice and subsequently diluted ten fold to the minimum required dilution (MRD) of the assay, in ABST buffer (acetate-buffered saline with 0.001% polysorbate 80, pH 6.0). MRD is defined as the minimum predilution of plasma sample needed in order to overcome matrix interference and to achieve acceptable performance during evaluation of validation parameters. For this two-step activity assay, MRD was established during method development at 1/10 as that was the minimum dilution at which plasma samples generated acceptable selectivity results (% recovery within 75–125%). Diluted samples were stored on ice until they were loaded onto the reaction plate.

Substrate, 4-MUS

The optimal concentration of the substrate, 4-MUS substrate (4-methylumbellifery α-L-iduronide-2-sulfate, C16H15O12S·2Na, molecular weight 477.33, Santa Cruz Biotechnologies, catalog no. sc-210122) was determined by side-by-side comparison of 1.2, 0.6, 0.3, 0.12, and 0.06 mg/mL concentrations in the same assay. Selection of 0.6 mg/mL was based on (a) the best dilutional linearity within the quantitative range of the assay (range of 50–1,000 ng/mL of AGT-182 plasma samples), (b) separation of signal amongst individual AGT-182 plasma samples ranging from 50 to 1,000 ng/mL, as well as (c) the highest signal/noise which was the ratio of the ULOQ at 1000 ng/mL over the blank plasma sample. These factors lead to the selection of 0.6 mg/mL as the optimal concentration of 4-MUS in this assay. At substrate concentration higher than 0.6 mg/mL, for example, 1.2 mg/mL, the assay background was elevated to 7,000–9,000 fluorescence units (FUs) which had suboptimal separation from the targeted LLOQ of the assay (data not shown).

α-L-Iduronidase

Recombinant human α-L-iduronidase (Shire) was expressed in stable human cell line (HT1080) using G418 selection. Production of IDUA was performed in a wave reactor seeded at 50,000 cells/mL, cultured for 10 days at 37 °C. Culture media was collected by perfusion and stored at 4 °C. At the end of the production run, the cell viability was maintained at ≥94%. The culture media of three wave runs were pooled and purified using a Ni-Sepharose Fast Flow column method. The fractions were pooled and dialyzed into 50 mM Na Acetate, 500 mM NaCl, pH 5.0 storage

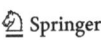

buffer. The purity of the final product was determined to be 94%.

Enzymatic Activity Assay

For the standard assay, reaction mixtures consisting of 10 μL of MRD-diluted plasma samples or controls and 20 μL of 0.6 mg/mL of substrate 4-MUS in substrate diluent (0.1 M sodium acetate, 10 mM lead acetate, 0.2% sodium azide, pH 5.0) were loaded in duplicates onto black polystyrene, non-treated plates (COSTAR, part no. 3915). Assay plates were immediately covered with foil sealers and placed in the 37 °C shaking incubator set at 350 RPM for 1 h. For the second reaction step, the IDUA working solution was prepared at 22 μg/mL in McIlvaine's buffer (0.4 M sodium phosphate dibasic, 0.2 M sodium citrate, 0.2% sodium azide, pH 4.5) and added at 45 μL per reaction to bring its final reaction concentration to 13.2 μg/mL. Plates were once again covered with foil sealers and placed in the 37 °C shaking incubator set at 350 RPM for 4 h. Reactions were stopped by the addition of 200 μL of Stop Solution (0.5 M sodium carbonate, 0.025% Triton X-100, pH 10.7). The final hydrolysis product, 4-MU, was quantitated against a standard curve prepared fresh in the Stop Solution using commercial 4-MU (MP Biomedicals, part no. 152475). 275 μL of each standard was loaded per well to match the final volume in the sample reaction wells. Fluorescence was measured at 365 nM (Ex), 450 nM (Em), 435 nM (Cutoff, defined as the wavelength for the filter at which the transmission is 50%) using a SpectraMax M5 (Molecular Devices) plate reader.

Calculation of Sample Activity

Calculations of sample activity were based on the mean of fluorescence unit of the duplicate wells extrapolated against the 4-MU standard curve. The 4-MU concentration of every sample was adjusted for the MRD as well as for any additional predilutions that the sample had been subjected to. Activity for unknown samples was calculated in nmol/h/mL using the following equation: Activity (nmol/h/mL) = [27.5 × (4-MU Result/1,000)] /1, where the denominator 1 represents the 1 h first step reaction time. Activity for the assay controls and some VSs was calculated in nmol/h/μg as appropriate for each particular validation parameter. This was done by dividing activity in nmol/h/mL by the μg/mL concentration of the control or the spiked VS. All activity results were corrected for the appropriate background; for example, the assay plasma controls were corrected for the unfortified plasma pool (the 0 ng/mL control), the validation selectivity samples were corrected for their matched unfortified individual plasma

samples, and unknown samples were corrected for their respective pre-dose or baseline samples.

Results

Method Development and Optimization

4-MU Standard Curve

The 4-MU standard curve was prepared by fortifying the assay Stop Solution with commercial 4-MU. The calibration curve range which was optimized to attain maximal sensitivity; the final quantitative range was from 31.25 to 4,000 nM.

I2S Reaction Time

The first step reaction involved catalysis of the substrate, 4-MUS, by I2S. According to previously published work (Voznyi et al. 2001), different laboratories carry out this step at either 1 or 4 h. We investigated whether 1 or 4 h constituted an optimal reaction time for this step. Figure 1a presents a comparison of activity for AGT-182-spiked samples after 1 or 4 h of first step. The data suggest that activity is in the linear

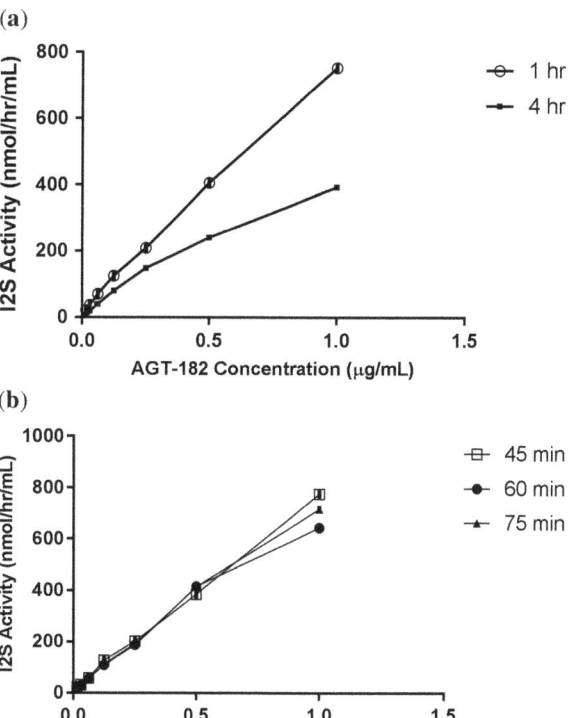

Fig. 1 Optimization of I2S reaction time. (**a**) A comparison of 1 and 4 h reactions times using plasma samples spiked with increasing concentrations of AGT-182. (**b**) Comparison of 45, 60, and 75 min to establish the acceptance limits of the 1 h reaction time

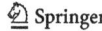 Springer

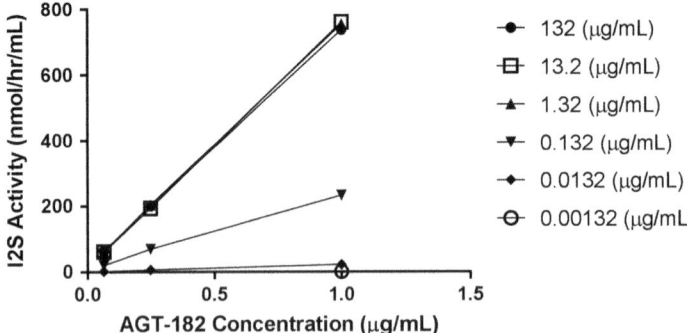

Fig. 2 Optimization of α-L-iduronidase. α-L-iduronidase was used in the second reaction step at ten-fold increasing concentrations ranging from 0.00132 to 132 μg/mL for the analysis of plasma samples fortified with AGT-182

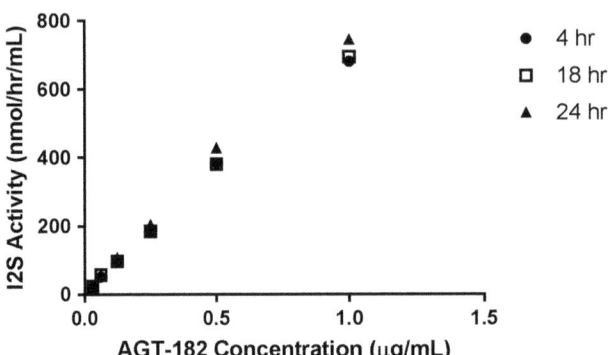

Fig. 3 Optimization of α-L-iduronidase reaction time. Evaluation of the second step reaction catalyzed by α-L-iduronidase and carried out for 4, 18, and 24 h using plasma samples containing varying concentrations of AGT-182

range after 1 h incubation but is diminished if the first step is carried out for 4 h potentially due to the exhaustion of the substrate. This comparison was repeated and confirmed in a separate experiment. Subsequently in a separate experiment, the first step reaction time was further optimized at the proximity of 1 h so that limits of this time window could be assessed. A comparison of 45, 60, and 75 min reaction times is shown in Fig. 1b; no significant difference was observed amongst the three conditions. It was therefore concluded that the first step could be carried out for anywhere within the 45–75 min window with optimal activity yields.

Optimization of α-L-Iduronidase Activity

To assess potency, efficiency, and maximal enzymatic activity of the Shire IDUA, this enzyme was evaluated at a multitude of concentrations which started with 132 μg/mL followed by serial ten-fold dilutions. The results are presented in Fig. 2 where activity in nmol/h/mL at each enzyme concentration is plotted against the concentration of AGT-182 in the plasma sample in μg/mL units. Data suggested that maximal enzymatic activity was achieved with IDUA concentrations ranging from 1.32 to 132 μg/

mL. Based on these results, 13.2 μg/mL which was ten folds higher than the activity saturation dose (1.32 μg/mL) was selected to avoid exhaustion of this enzyme during the second step reaction. In a separate but similar assay, the IDUA used in this study was compared to IDUA from a commercial source (R&D Systems, Minneapolis, MN). The activity and potency of IDUA from the two sources were shown to be identical when used at equal concentrations (data not shown).

Optimization of IDUA Reaction Time

The second step reaction catalyzed by IDUA is commonly run for 24 h according to published data (Voznyi et al. 2001). This makes for a 2-day assay. For efficiency purposes, shorter incubation times were evaluated to determine the feasibility of a 1-day assay. An activity assay was performed with three identical sets of AGT-182-fortified plasma samples in which the second step reaction was carried out for 4, 18, and 24 h, respectively. The data are presented in Fig. 3 and demonstrate that the activity difference between a 24 h reaction versus either 4 or 18 h reaction ranges from zero to 11%, and that the activity

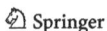

yields are generally similar for all three reaction times. Based on these results, a 4 h incubation time was selected so as to allow for the completion of the two-step assay in 1 day.

Method Validation

Accuracy and Precision

Inter- and intra-assay accuracy and precision were assessed in six independent runs with three sets of each VS level per run, by two operators using VSs prepared by spiking AGT-182 into qualified human plasma pool at five levels which included 50, 100, 400, 800, and 1,000 ng/mL for LLOQ, low, medium, high, and ULOQ, respectively. VS activity values were reported in nmol/h/µg and were each corrected for the endogenous plasma pool activity. The calculation of inter- and intra-assay precision was based on the ANOVA analysis method of DeSilva et al. (2003). Results are presented in Table 1 and show that relative error (RE) for all five VSs was in the targeted acceptance range of ±20%. RE was calculated using the following equation:

$$\%RE = \frac{\text{Measured Activity of Individual VS} - \text{Mean Activity of A\&P VSs}}{\text{Mean Activity of A\&P VSs}} \times 100$$

where the mean of all VSs assessed in the accuracy and precision runs was used as reference to establish the expected activity value in nmol/h/µg. The range of specific activity for AGT-182 based on accuracy and precision data was 524.0–655.0 nmol/h/µg. The range of specific activity based on all data obtained during method development and validation was 517.3–688.8 nmol/h/µg. The total error was calculated by adding the RE absolute value to the inter-assay CV; it met the targeted specification of ±30%. Inter-

and intra-assay CVs were <20% for all VSs and met the precision acceptance criteria.

Selectivity and Dilutional Linearity

Selectivity was evaluated by spiking ten individual human K_2EDTA plasma samples from normal healthy donors with AGT-182 at low and high levels. The low selectivity spike level was 70 ng/mL to position it between the LLOQ and the LQC of the assay; the high spike level was 800 ng/mL. The qualified plasma pool was also spiked with AGT-182 at the same levels as baseline control. The endogenous I2S activity in all unfortified samples was also evaluated. Percent recovery was determined as the ratio of measured activity in nmol/h/µg over expected activity using the following equation:

$$\%Recovery = (\text{Measured Activity of Individual Plasma}/\\\text{Expected Activity}) \times 100$$

Where Expected Activity = (Activity of Unspiked Sample) + (Total Expected Activity for the AGT-182 spike level of 70 or 800 ng/mL)

Expected Activity for the AGT-182 spike level of 70 or 800 ng/mL = (Reference mean activity of positive controls from accuracy and precision runs in nmol/h/µg) × 0.07(for 70 ng/mL) or 0.8 (for 800 ng/mL)

All ten individual plasma samples met the target selectivity recovery acceptance criteria of 75–125% at both high and low spike levels.

To evaluate linearity of dilution, an ultrahigh sample was prepared from the qualified plasma pool freshly spiked with 30 µg/mL of AGT-182. This sample was serially two-fold diluted from 1/2 through 1/ 20,480 in the matrix pool,

Table 1 Method accuracy and precision

	LLOQ 50 ng/mL	LQC 100 ng/mL	MQC 400 ng/mL	HQC 800 ng/mL	ULOQ 1,000 ng/mL
Mean activity (nmol/h/µg)	628.9	655.0	604.1	553.3	524.0
%RE[a]	4.1	8.4	0.0	−8.4	−13.3
Intra-assay precision (%CV)	7.8	7.1	0.8	1.9	1.3
Inter-assay precision (%CV)	10.1	8.7	9.0	7.3	7.1
|RE| + inter-assay CV	11.9	15.5	0.8	10.3	14.6

Inter- and intra-assay precision were evaluated by spiking the qualified plasma pool with AGT-182 at 50, 100, 400, 800, and 1,000 ng/mL for LLOQ, low, medium, high, and ULOQ, respectively. The resulting activities in nmol/h/µg for each of these validation samples were adjusted by the activity of unspiked plasma pool. The mean in nmol/h/µg of all validation samples was used to establish the expected activity value. Relative error (RE) was calculated as the percent difference between measured activity of individual validation sample and the theoretical value (mean activity of A&P)

[a] Mean of all A&P activity, 604.1 nmol/h/µg, was used to establish the expected activity for the calculation of relative error

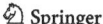

subsequently subjected to the MRD, and finally analyzed in the activity assay. The recovery of linearity samples was assessed as follows:

$$\%Recovery = (Mean\ Activity\ of\ the\ Dilution\ Sample/\ Expected\ Activity) \times 100$$

Where Expected Activity = (Activity of Plasma Pool) + (Activity value associated with the Ultrahigh Sample/ Dilution Factor)

Activity value associated with the Ultrahigh Sample = (Reference mean activity of positive controls based on accuracy and precision runs in nmol/h/μg) × 30

In the above formulae, the dilution factor includes the MRD of assay. Linearity samples with in-range nominal concentrations (expected concentration between 50 and 1,000 ng/mL) produced recoveries that ranged from 100 to 116% and met the targeted acceptance criteria of 75–125%. These data established linearity of sample dilution for up to 1/20,480 (data not shown).

Discussion

Through a series of optimizations and modifications, we were able to improve the I2S two-step enzymatic activity assay from a 2-day format into a 1-day assay which can be completed in less than 6 h and is more robust. The resulting two-step enzymatic activity assay is specific towards I2S as the assay substrate could only be hydrolyzed by I2S. Additionally, this assay leads to complete hydrolysis of the starting substrate; this feature helps reduce variability across runs and across multiple sample measurements.

Application of the activity assay in regulated studies requires full validation of the method, and since the enzymatic activity was intended for pharmacokinetic assessment, it was important that method validation followed the FDA regulatory guidance for validation of quantitative LBAs as closely as possible. The absence of a typical LBA calibration curve to allow for extrapolation of sample values in the same concentration units of ng/mL or μg/mL as used for spiking the VSs was a significant challenge. We devised a methodology to establish the expected (spike) values in activity units of nmol/h/mL or nmol/h/μg based on the mean of measured activity values for VSs. This allowed for the calculation of the accuracy as percent of measured over expected values in each validation run. Subsequently method validation was conducted in accordance with the agency guidance as part of which, validation parameters including accuracy and preci-

sion, selectivity, dilutional linearity, and stability were assessed using the above approach. All validation parameters successfully passed the acceptance criteria. A summary of method development, optimization, and validation results were presented in this paper.

Enzymatic activity assays have become instrumental in the assessment of pharmacokinetics, pharmacodynamics, efficacy, and biofunction of ERTs. Optimization of such assays into more specific, robust, efficient, and faster methods will improve the quality of the PK data as well as have cost saving impact.

Acknowledgements Mitra Azadeh, Luying Pan, and Yongchang Qiu are full time employees of Shire. Ruben Boado is a full time employee of ArmaGen. We thank Eurofins Pharma Bioanalytics Services, St Charles, MO, USA, contracted by Shire to perform validation of the two-step activity method, for their services. We also thank the Shire Discovery Therapeutic Group for providing the IDUA.

Synopsis

Effective optimization resulted in an I2S enzymatic activity assay which is rapid, more specific, more robust, highly reproducible, and hence better suited for application in clinical or nonclinical studies.

Compliance with Ethics Guidelines

Conflict of Interest

Mitra Azadeh, Luying Pan, Yongchang Qiu, and Ruben Boado declare that they have no conflict of interest.

Informed Consent/Animal Rights

This article does not contain any studies with human or animal subjects performed by any of the authors.

Funding

Funding for this work was provided by Shire.

Author Contributions

Mitra Azadeh was responsible for the design, planning, conduct, data analysis, and reporting of the work described in this publication; she also drafted this article. Luying Pan, Yongchang Qiu, Ruben Boado, and Mitra Azadeh equally contributed to the interpretation of the data and critical revisions of the article for important intellectual content.

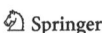

References

Boado RJ et al (2014) Insulin receptor antibody-iduronate 2-sulfatase fusion protein; pharmacokinetics, anti-drug antibody, and safety pharmacology in rhesus monkeys. Biotechnol Bioeng 111(11): 2317–2324

DeSilva B et al (2003) Recommendations for bioanalytical method validation of ligand-binding assays to support pharmacokinetics assessment of macromolecules. Pharm Res 20(11):1885–1990

Hopwood JJ (1979) α-L-Iduronidase, β-D-glucuronidase, and sulfo-L-iduronate 2-sulfatase: preparation and characterization of radioactive substrate from heparin. Carbohydr Res 69:203–216

Inoue H et al (1982) Fluorometric determination of arylsulfatase A and B activities. Chem Pharm Bull 30(11):4140–4143

Johnson BA et al (2013) Diagnosing lysosomal storage disorders: mucopolysaccharidosis type II. Current Prot Hum Genetics. doi: 10.1002/0471142905.hg1714s79

Lu JZ et al (2010) Genetic engineering of a biofunctional fusion protein with iduronate-2-sulfatase. Bioconjug Chem 21:151–156

Muenzer J et al (2006) A phase II/III clinical study of enzyme replacement therapy with idursulfase in mucopolysaccharidosis II (Hunter syndrome). Genet Med 8(8):465–473

Muenzer J et al (2007) A phase I/II clinical trial of enzyme replacement therapy in mucopolysaccharidosis II (Hunter syndrome). Mol Gen Metab 90:329–337

Tolun AA et al (2012) A novel fluorometric enzyme analysis method for Hunter syndrome using dried blood spots. Mol Genetics Met 105: 519–521

Voznyi YV et al (2001) A fluorimetric enzyme assay for the diagnosis of MPS II (Hunter disease). J Inhert Metab Dis 24:675–680

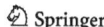

JIMD Reports
DOI 10.1007/8904_2017_35

RESEARCH REPORT

An Unexplained Congenital Disorder of Glycosylation-II in a Child with Neurohepatic Involvement, Hypercholesterolemia and Hypoceruloplasminemia

Pier Luigi Calvo · Marco Spada · Ivana Rabbone ·
Michele Pinon · Francesco Porta · Fabio Cisarò ·
Stefania Reggiani · Angelo B. Cefalù ·
Luisella Sturiale · Domenico Garozzo ·
Dirk J. Lefeber · Jaak Jaeken

Received: 11 January 2017 /Revised: 28 May 2017 /Accepted: 31 May 2017 /Published online: 23 June 2017
© SSIEM and Springer-Verlag Berlin Heidelberg 2017

Abstract We report on a 12-year-old adopted boy with psychomotor disability, absence seizures, and normal brain MRI. He showed increased (but initially, at 5 months, normal) serum cholesterol, increased alkaline phosphatases, transiently increased transaminases and hypoceruloplasminemia with normal serum and urinary copper. Blood levels of immunoglobulins, haptoglobin, antithrombin, and factor XI were normal. A type 2 serum transferrin isoelectrofocusing and hypoglycosylation of apoCIII pointed to a combined N- and O-glycosylation defect. Neither CDG

panel analysis with 79 CDG-related genes, nor whole exome sequencing revealed the cause of this CDG. Whole genome sequencing was not performed since the biological parents of this adopted child were not available.

Abbreviations

ALP	Alkaline phosphatase
apoCIII	Apolipoprotein CIII
AST, ALT	Serum transaminases
CDG	Congenital disorders of glycosylation
CK	Creatine kinase
GGT	Gamma glutamyltransferase
IEF	Isoelectrofocusing
MALDI-TOF	Matrix-assisted laser desorption/ionization-time of flight
Tf	Serum transferrin

Communicated by: Eva Morava, MD PhD

P. L. Calvo (✉) · M. Pinon · F. Cisarò · S. Reggiani
Pediatric Gastroenterology Unit, Department of Pediatrics, Azienda Ospedaliera-Universitaria Città della Salute e della Scienza di Torino, University of Torino, Piazza Polonia 94, Torino 10126, Italy
e-mail: pcalvo@cittadellasalute.to.it

M. Spada · I. Rabbone · F. Porta
Department of Pediatrics, Azienda Ospedaliera-Universitaria Città della Salute e della Scienza di Torino, University of Torino, Torino, Italy

A. B. Cefalù
Department of Biomedicine, Internal Medicine and Medical Specialties (DIBIMIS), University of Palermo, Palermo, Italy

L. Sturiale · D. Garozzo
CNR Institute for Polymers Composites and Biomaterials, Catania, Italy

D. J. Lefeber
Translational Metabolic Laboratory, Department of Neurology, Radboudumc, Nijmegen, The Netherlands

J. Jaeken
Department of Development and Regeneration, Centre for Metabolic Disease, University Hospital Gasthuisberg, KU Leuven, Leuven, Belgium

Introduction

Congenital disorders of glycosylation (CDG) are due to defects in the glycoprotein and glycolipid glycan synthesis and attachment. Glycoprotein glycosylation defects comprise disorders of N-glycosylation, O-glycosylation, and combined N- and O-glycosylation disorders (Jaeken and Morava 2016; Wolfe and Krasnewich 2013). Defective N-glycosylation is usually diagnosed by finding an abnormal serum transferrin (Tf) isoelectrofocusing (IEF) pattern (Jaeken et al. 1984). A type 1 pattern points to a defect in glycan assembly (CDG-I; cytosolic or ER defect), and a type 2 pattern to a defect in glycan remodelling (CDG-II; Golgi defect). The diagnosis of some (mucin type 1)

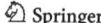

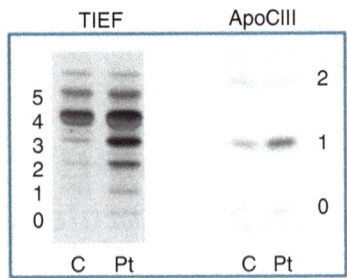
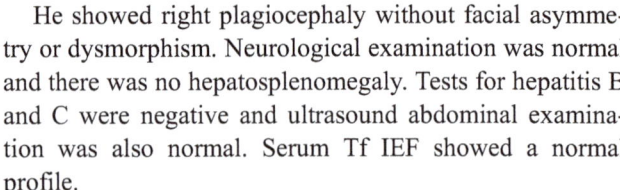

Fig. 1 Transferrin isofocusing for analysis of protein N-glycosylation showed increased disialo- and trisialotransferrin; isofocusing of apoCIII for analysis of mucin type O-glycosylation showed increased apoCIII-1 and decreased ApoCIII-2

O-glycosylation defects can be made by IEF of serum apolipoprotein CIII (apoCIII), showing a cathodal shift (Wopereis et al. 2003). The next step in the diagnosis, after excluding a protein variant and secondary hypoglycosylation, is mutation analysis of a panel of glycosylation genes. If this analysis reveals a normal result, whole exome sequencing should be performed and, if necessary, whole genome sequencing (Matthijs et al. 2013).

We report on a patient with a neurological presentation, transient biochemical liver involvement and other serum abnormalities, particularly hypercholesterolemia and hypoceruloplasminemia. Further investigation showed a type 2 serum Tf IEF and hyposialylation of apoCIII (Fig. 1). Neither CDG panel mutation analysis with 79 genes involved in CDG nor whole exome sequencing could reveal the cause of this CDG-IIx. Whole genome sequencing was not performed since the biological parents of this adopted patient were not available.

Case Report

This 12-year-old boy was adopted at the age of 8 months because his mother had intellectual disability. His birth weight was 3.500 g. He came to our attention at 5 months (weight 6.500 g, between 10 and 25th percentiles; length 67 cm, 50th percentile; head circumference 42 cm, 25th percentile) because of increased serum transaminases (AST: 100 U/L [normal: <41], ALT: 97 U/L [normal: <41]) and gamma glutamyltransferase (GGT) (286 U/L [normal: <71 IU/L]). Serum bilirubin, INR, aPTT, albumin, total and LDL cholesterol, and triglycerides were normal. Serum biliary acids were mildly increased (15.3 μmol/L; normal range 0–10). Alkaline phosphatase (ALP) levels were highly increased: 5,613 U/L (normal range 300–850 U/L). Serum α1-antitrypsin (serum dosage, immunoelectrophoresis, and genetic test), autoantibodies (ANA, ASMA, LKM, AMA), celiac disease antibody tests, plasma amino acids, and urinary organic acids were normal.

He showed right plagiocephaly without facial asymmetry or dysmorphism. Neurological examination was normal and there was no hepatosplenomegaly. Tests for hepatitis B and C were negative and ultrasound abdominal examination was also normal. Serum Tf IEF showed a normal profile.

At 1 year, neurological examination was still normal. Serum transaminases had nearly normalized (AST 61, ALT 31 UI/L). GGT was normal as was creatine kinase (CK), but alkaline phosphatase was still high (1,574 U/L). Alkaline phosphatase isoenzyme analysis showed a 14% hepatic component (normal range 1–31%), a 76% bone component (normal range 62–100%), and a 9% biliary component (normal range 1–7%). Serum 25-OH vitamin D and 1,25-OH vitamin D were normal. His psychomotor development was relatively slow: he spoke his first words at 15 months and walked without support at 18 months.

At 22 months, a re-evaluation showed stable liver values and ALP profile, but a significant increase in cholesterol (total: 332 mg/dL, LDL-C: 240 mg/dL; HDL-C: 69 mg/dL) with persistently normal triglycerides (64 mg/dL), a normal apolipoprotein profile, INR, aPTT, antithrombin, factor XI. Serum copper was normal but ceruloplasmin was decreased (9 mg/dL [normal range: 20–40]). Twenty-four hour cupruria was repeatedly normal (<40 μg/24 h) and ATP7B mutation analysis was negative. Repeat IEF of serum Tf then showed a type 2 profile (increases in trisialo-, disialo-, monosialo-, and asialoTf) (Fig. 1). A Tf protein variant was excluded after neuraminidase treatment. Serum Tf glycan analysis using matrix-assisted laser desorption/ionization-time of flight (MALDI-TOF) showed hyposialylation and mild hypogalactosylation (increase of a monosialo biantennary glycan and an abnormal peak corresponding to a monosialo-, monogalacto-biantennary glycan), (not shown). Also IEF of serum ApoCIII) showed hyposialylation (increased apoCIII-1 and decreased ApoCIII-2) (Fig. 1). Neither CDG panel mutation analysis with 79 genes involved in CDG nor whole exome sequencing revealed pathogenic variants. Whole genome sequencing was not performed since the biological parents of this child were not available.

His further evaluation showed mild developmental and speech disability. Brain MRI at 3½ and 8 years was normal. Physical examination, including liver and spleen, was normal. He attended school with a support teacher. At 8 years, he had repeated episodes of absence seizures with a pathological EEG that responded to levetiracetam.

He showed a progressive normalization of serum transaminases and GGT (last examination at 12 years: AST 33 U/L, ALT 15 U/L, GGT 10 IU/L), but persistently high ALP (957 U/L) and cholesterol levels (at 6 years: total cholesterol 351 mg/dL, LDL cholesterol 264 dL, HDL cholesterol 68 mg/dL).

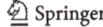

Targeted resequencing of candidate genes (i.e. *LDLR, APOB, PCSK9, LDLRAP1, ABCG5/8*) was carried out by a NGS customized panel using the Ion PGM Sequencer. No variants with potential pathogenic effects were detected in the above-mentioned candidate genes. Also, in the WES data, these genes were looked at but no mutations found.

Serum ceruloplasmin remained low (7 mg/dL) with normal cupruria (<40 μg/24 h). Serum 25-OH vitamin D (5.3 ng/mL; normal range: 9–37) became subnormal despite oral supplementation. Serum levels of free T4, TSH, haptoglobin, IgG, IgA, and IgM were normal. Cholestyramine treatment, started at 8 years, led to a significant decrease in cholesterol levels (at 12 years: total cholesterol 220, LDL cholesterol 164, HDL cholesterol 42 mg/dL). A recent fibroscan showed no liver fibrosis.

Discussion

The patient discussed herein shows neurological involvement (learning difficulties and epilepsy) as well as biochemical evidence of a liver disorder. This is associated with a combined deficiency of N- and O-glycosylation, as shown by the type 2 pattern of serum Tf IEF and the hypoglycosylation pattern of serum apoCIII. Known CDG with a combined N- and O-glycosylation deficiency was excluded by CDG panel analysis and whole exome sequencing. A particular feature of this patient was his hypercholesterolemia. Since his biological parents could not be investigated, isolated familial hypercholesterolemia could not be excluded. The fact that at 5 months serum cholesterol was still normal may be in favor of an association with his CDG. Moreover, targeted resequencing of candidate genes of autosomal dominant and recessive hypercholesterolemias did not reveal either known pathogenic variants or novel variants of uncertain significance. Hypocholesterolemia is a well-known feature of PMM2-CDG and other CDG-I (Stibler et al. 1991; Weinstein et al. 2005; Tegtmeyer et al. 2014). It is usually attributed to a decrease in the cholesterol binding proteins apo A and apo B. Hypercholesterolemia is an exceptional feature in CDG. It has recently been reported in CCDC115-CDG (Jansen et al. 2016a) and TMEM199-CDG (Calvo et al. 2008; Jansen et al. 2016b), combined N- and O-glycosylation disorders of Golgi homeostasis. No explanation was provided for the hypercholesterolemia in these patients. Both these disorders, as well as the recently reported ATP6AP1-CDG (Jansen et al. 2016c), also showed hypoceruloplasminemia as does our patient. However, these patients also had hypocupremia and some had a mild increase in hepatic liver copper, differently from our patient. Hypoceruloplasminemia is not a recent finding in CDG; in fact, it has been reported in CDG-I, particularly

PMM2-CDG, as one of the many glycoprotein abnormalities characteristic of these CDG (Harrison and Miller 1992; Henri et al. 1997; Heywood et al. 2016). However, the other investigated glycoproteins were normal in our patient. Mandato et al. (2006) also reported on four patients with subclinical liver involvement, a type 2 serum Tf IEF, and hypoceruloplasminemia. Differently from our patient, they did not have any neurological involvement, patients 1 and 2 also showed decreased serum copper and patients 3 and 4 a persistent decrease of multiple coagulation factors. The CDG type(s) in their patients and in our patient remain(s) to be determined.

Acknowledgements The authors wish to thank Mrs. Barbara Wade for her linguistic advice.

Take Home Message

Hypercholesterolemia and hypoceruloplasminemia, in a child with neurohepatic involvement, could be due to a congenital disorder of glycosylation, sometimes, as in this case, still unexplained.

Pier Luigi Calvo, Jaak Jaeken conceptualized and designed the study and drafted the initial manuscript.

Marco Spada, Ivana Rabbone, Michele Pinon, Francesco Porta, Fabio Cisarò, Stefania Reggiani, Angelo B. Cefalù, L. Sturiale, D. Garozzo, Dirk J. Lefeber conceptualized and designed the study and reviewed and revised the manuscript. All authors approved the final manuscript as submitted and agreed to be accountable for all aspects of the work.

Communicated by: Pier Luigi Calvo.

Competing interest: none declared.

Funding source: no funding.

Financial disclosure: no financial relationships relevant to this article to disclose.

Ethics approval: yes.

Patient consent statement: obtained.

References

Calvo PL, Pagliardini S, Baldi M et al (2008) Long-standing mild hypertransaminasaemia caused by congenital disorder of glycosylation (CDG) type IIx. J Inherit Metab Dis 31(Suppl 2): S437–S440

Harrison H, Miller K (1992) Multiple serum protein abnormalities in carbohydrate-deficient glycoprotein syndrome: pathognomonic finding of two-dimensional electrophoresis. Clin Chem 38:1390–1392

Henri H, Tissot JD, Messerli B et al (1997) Microheterogeneity of serum glycoproteins and their liver precursors in patients with carbohydrate-deficient glycoprotein syndrome type I: apparent deficiencies in clusterin and serum amyloid P. J Lab Clin Med 129:412–421

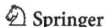

Heywood WE, Bliss E, Mills P et al (2016) Global serum glycoform profiling for the investigation of dystroglycanopathies § congenital disorders of glycosylation. Mol Genet Metab Rep 7:55–62

Jaeken J, Morava E (2016) Congenital disorders of glycosylation, dolichol and glycosylphosphatidylinositol metabolism. In: Saudubray JM, van den Berghe G, Walter JH (eds) Inborn metabolic diseases – diagnosis and treatment, 6th edn. Springer, Berlin

Jaeken J, van Eijk HG, van der Heul C et al (1984) Sialic acid-deficient serum and cerebrospinal fluid transferrin in a newly recognized genetic syndrome. Clin Chim Acta 144:245–247

Jansen JC, Cirak S, van Scherpenzeel M et al (2016a) CCDC115 deficiency causes a disorder of Golgi homeostasis with abnormal protein glycosylation. Am J Hum Genet 98:310–321

Jansen JC, Timal S, van Scherpenzeel M et al (2016b) TMEM199 deficiency is a disorder of Golgi homeostasis characterized by elevated transaminases, alkaline phosphatase, and cholesterol and abnormal glycosylation. Am J Hum Genet 98:322–330

Jansen EJR, Timal S, Ryan M et al (2016c) ATP6AP1 deficiency causes an immunodeficiency with hepatopathy, cognitive impairment and abnormal protein glycosylation. Nat Commun 7:11600. doi:10.1038/ncomms11600

Mandato C, Brive L, Miura Y et al (2006) Cryptogenic liver disease in four children: a novel congenital disorder of glycosylation. Pediatr Res 59:293–298

Matthijs G, Rymen D, Millón MB et al (2013) Approaches to homozygosity mapping and exome sequencing for the identification of novel types of CDG. Glycoconj J 30:67–76

Stibler H, Jaeken J, Kristiansson B (1991) Biochemical characteristics and diagnosis of the carbohydrate-deficient glycoprotein syndrome. Acta Paediatr Scand Suppl 375:21–31

Tegtmeyer LC, Rust S, van Scherpenzeel M et al (2014) Multiple phenotypes in phosphoglucomutase 1 deficiency. N Engl J Med 370:533–542

Weinstein M, Schollen E, Matthijs G et al (2005) CDG-IL: an infant with a novel mutation in the ALG9 gene and additional phenotypic features. Am J Hum Genet 136A:194–197

Wolfe LA, Krasnewich D (2013) Congenital disorders of glycosylation and intellectual disability. Dev Disabil Res Rev 17:211–225

Wopereis S, Grünewald S, Morava E et al (2003) Apolipoprotein C-III isofocusing in the diagnosis of genetic defects in O-glycan biosynthesis. Clin Chem 49:1839–1845

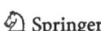

JIMD Reports
DOI 10.1007/8904_2017_37

RESEARCH REPORT

Peripheral Neuropathy, Episodic Rhabdomyolysis, and Hypoparathyroidism in a Patient with Mitochondrial Trifunctional Protein Deficiency

Peter van Vliet · Annelies E. Berden ·
Mojca K. M. van Schie · Jaap A. Bakker ·
Christian Heringhaus · Irenaeus F. M. de Coo ·
Mirjam Langeveld · Marielle A. Schroijen ·
M. Sesmu Arbous

Received: 26 February 2017 / Revised: 23 May 2017 / Accepted: 07 June 2017 / Published online: 07 July 2017
© SSIEM and Springer-Verlag Berlin Heidelberg 2017

Abstract A combination of unexplained peripheral neuropathy, hypoparathyroidism, and the inability to cope with metabolic stress could point to a rare inborn error of metabolism, such as mitochondrial trifunctional protein (MTP) deficiency.

Here, we describe a 20-year-old woman who was known since childhood with axonal motor sensory polyneuropathy of unknown origin. She presented with progressive dyspnoea, and increased muscle weakness, preceded by 6 days of fever, vomiting, and diarrhoea. Laboratory testing showed rhabdomyolysis, and hypocalcaemia with low parathyroid levels. The patient was intubated because of respiratory insufficiency and a viral and bacterial pneumonia was diagnosed. She was discharged after 16 days of admission. Metabolic screening, performed at the time of rhabdomyolysis, showed increased concentrations of long-chain 3-hydroxyacyl carnitine species, together with elevated urinary excretion of 3-hydroxy dicarboxylic acids. Decreased activity of long-chain 3-hydroxyacyl-CoA dehydrogenase and long-chain 3-ketoacyl-CoA thiolase in peripheral lymphocytes and fibroblasts confirmed a MTP deficiency. Sequence analysis of the *HADHB* gene showed two heterozygous variants: c.209+1G>C (splicing defect) and c.980T>C (p.Leu327Leu). When the acylcarnitine profile was repeated after the episode of rhabdomyolysis had resolved it showed no abnormalities.

Our case illustrates a cluster of peripheral neuropathy, episodic rhabdomyolysis, and hypoparathyroidism in a patient with MTP deficiency caused by mutations in the *HADHB* gene. It stresses the importance of performing metabolic screening when patients are most symptomatic, as normal results can be found at times when no metabolic stress is present. Screening is relatively easy and timely diagnosis has important implications for treatment.

Communicated by: Manuel Schiff

Peter van Vliet and Annelies E. Berden contributed equally to this work.

Electronic supplementary material: The online version of this chapter (doi:10.1007/8904_2017_37) contains supplementary material, which is available to authorized users.

P. van Vliet (✉) · M. S. Arbous
Department of Intensive Care Medicine, Leiden University Medical Center, Leiden, The Netherlands
e-mail: p.van_vliet@yahoo.com

A. E. Berden · M. A. Schroijen
Department of Internal Medicine, Leiden University Medical Center, Leiden, The Netherlands

M. K. M. van Schie
Department of Neurology, Leiden University Medical Center, Leiden, The Netherlands

J. A. Bakker
Department of Clinical Chemistry, Leiden University Medical Center, Leiden, The Netherlands

C. Heringhaus
Emergency Department, Leiden University Medical Center, Leiden, The Netherlands

I. F. M. de Coo
Department of Neurology, Erasmus University Medical Center, Rotterdam, The Netherlands

M. Langeveld
Department of Endocrinology and Metabolism, Academic Medical Centre, University of Amsterdam, Amsterdam, The Netherlands

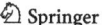

Introduction

Mitochondrial trifunctional protein (MTP) is a multi-enzyme complex which catalyses the last three steps of the β-oxidation of long-chain fatty acids in mitochondria. MTP is a hetero-octamer consisting of four α-subunits and four β-subunits that harbour enzyme activity of long-chain 3-hydroxyacyl-CoA dehydrogenase (LCHAD), long-chain enoyl-CoA hydratase (LCEH), and long-chain 3-ketoacyl-CoA thiolase (LCKAT). MTP deficiency and isolated LCHAD deficiency are clinically indistinguishable. MTP deficiency is caused by mutations in the genes *HADHA* and *HADHB*, encoding the α- and the β-subunits, respectively, resulting in decreased enzyme activity of all three enzymes, whereas the majority of patients of European origin with isolated LCHAD deficiency are homozygous for a common mutation in the *HADHA* gene (Spiekerkoetter et al. 2003a; Brackett et al. 1995).

MTP deficiency is a rare disorder; during a 6-year period only 11 patients were identified out of 1.2 million newborns screened in the routine neonatal screening program in Germany (Sander et al. 2005). Since the start of screening in the Netherlands in 2007, 8 patients with MTP deficiency have been identified, which corresponds to an annual incidence of 1 patient per 200,000 newborns (personal communication). MTP deficiency has a heterogeneous clinical presentation, with disease severity depending on both residual enzyme activity and the exposure to stress (Morris and Spiekerkoetter 2016). Patients with severe deficiency present with severe neonatal disease, characterized by cardiomyopathy, arrhythmias, (hepatic) encephalopathy, and early death. Another phenotype, resembling that of patients with isolated LCHAD deficiency, is characterized by recurrent episodes of hypoketotic hypoglycaemia that are generally induced by illness and prolonged fasting. A milder phenotype, with late-onset (juvenile/adolescent) type of disease, presents with myopathy, episodic rhabdomyolysis, peripheral neuropathy, and retinopathy (Morris and Spiekerkoetter 2016; Boutron et al. 2011; Spiekerkoetter et al. 2003b). Although there is no strict genotype–phenotype correlation, mutations in *HADHB* gene are primarily associated with the severe neonatal disease form, whereas mutations in the *HADHA* gene associate with all disease phenotypes (Boutron et al. 2011). Because MTP deficiency is a rare disease with a highly variable clinical presentation, establishing the diagnosis can be challenging.

Here we report a 20-year-old patient with MTP deficiency who was diagnosed after an episode of severe rhabdomyolysis and respiratory weakness requiring mechanical ventilation, following a pneumonia. Interestingly, a concomitant diagnosis of hypoparathyroidism was made.

Case Presentation

A 20-year-old woman presented to the emergency department with progressive dyspnoea and difficulty swallowing since 2 days. These symptoms were preceded by 6 days of fever, abdominal pain, vomiting, and diarrhoea. She also reported increased muscle weakness with difficulty moving her arms and she had not been able to walk for days. In the previous weeks she suffered from a common cold and a persistent cough.

Her medical history included slowly progressive distal weakness and sensory deficits (gnostic more than vital) of the lower extremities, pes cavus, areflexia, and electromyographic signs of an axonal motor sensory polyneuropathy (Supplementary Table 1). This was attributed to hereditary motor and sensory neuropathy (HMSN), although this diagnosis was not confirmed on a molecular level. Later obtained medical history also revealed shuddering attacks with reduced consciousness, which started from 40 days after birth. A concomitant hypocalcaemia, caused by hypoparathyroidism, was interpreted as the possible explanation for these attacks. The patient used active vitamin D for a short-term, which was discontinued for unknown reasons. In recent years she experienced muscle pain and cramps with exercise and occasionally had red urine. Her parents were non-consanguineous and from North-African descent. Both parents and her younger brother and sister were healthy and none had signs of peripheral neuropathy.

In the emergency room the patient was tachycardic (105 beats per minute), breathing was shallow at a rate of 25 breaths per minute, accompanied by the use of accessory muscles of respiration and difficulty speaking, but with sufficient oxygenation without oxygen support. There was upper quadrant abdominal tenderness. Neurological examination revealed weakness of neck extensors and -flexors with head drop, and symmetrical weakness of proximal and distal muscles of upper and lower extremities. Muscle strength was 'Medical research council' (MRC)-scale 3/3 of proximal arm muscles, 4/4 of distal arm muscles, 3/3 of proximal leg muscles, 4/4 of foot extensors, and 1/1 of foot flexors. Sensory testing revealed hypoesthesia of the lower extremities, and absent vibration sense in all extremities. Deep tendon reflexes were absent, corresponding with previous examinations.

Laboratory testing showed severe rhabdomyolysis with creatine kinase (CK) of 193,936 U/L (normal range: 0–145 U/L). Aspartate aminotransferase (ASAT) was 2,781 U/L (0–31 U/L), alanine aminotransferase (ALAT) was 791 U/L (0–34 U/L), and lactate dehydrogenase (LDH) was 3,583 U/L (0–247 U/L), with otherwise normal liver enzyme tests. Corrected calcium was 1.48 mmol/L (2.15–2.55 mmol/L), and anorganic phosphate 2.41 mmol/L

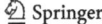

(0.90–1.50 mmol/L), with otherwise normal electrolyte levels and renal function. Parathyroid hormone (PTH) level was 0.6 pmol/L (0.7–8.0 pmol/L), and 25-OH-vitamin D level was 17 nmol/L (50–250 nmol/L). Complete blood count and coagulation tests were normal. Chest X-ray and abdominal ultrasonography showed no relevant abnormalities.

The patient was admitted to the intensive care unit, where intravenous hydration was started for severe rhabdomyolysis and calcium was supplemented. Because of the severe rhabdomyolysis, plasma, and urine samples were collected for metabolic screening. On the second day of admission the patient was intubated because of respiratory insufficiency. Shortly hereafter she developed fever and was treated with broad-spectrum antibiotics for community acquired pneumonia. Oseltamivir was added after molecular diagnostics revealed Influenza B RNA. Sputum cultures showed *Staphylococcus aureus* and *Moraxella catarrhalis* and antibiotics were narrowed-down accordingly. After 9 days the patient was extubated and 2 days later she was transferred to the neurology ward. Muscle strength normalized to pre-admission levels, and she was discharged after 16 days of admission. Laboratory testing 4 weeks later revealed complete normalization of aminotransferases and a still slightly elevated CK of 580 U/L.

Fourteen weeks after the first presentation the patient suffered another episode of rhabdomyolysis that followed two weeks of diarrhoea and several days without oral intake, most likely caused by a viral gastroenteritis. Laboratory testing revealed a CK of 28,660 U/L, ASAT of 416 U/L, ALAT of 125 U/L, LDH of 801 U/L, corrected calcium of 1.74 mmol/L, and PTH level of 0.6 pmol/L. Intravenous hydration was started for rhabdomyolysis, and the hypoparathyroidism was treated with intravenous and oral calcium supplementation, as well as alfacalcidol. She quickly recovered and was discharged after 7 days.

During the second admission the metabolic screening results became available and showed increased concentrations of long-chain 3-hydroxyacyl carnitine species, together with elevated urinary excretion of 3-hydroxy dicarboxylic acids. Following this, activity of enzymes involved in the β-oxidation of long-chain fatty acids was measured in peripheral lymphocytes and fibroblasts

(Table 1). Both LCHAD and LKAT activity were strongly reduced, pointing towards a MTP deficiency. Sequence analysis of the *HADHB* gene showed two heterozygous variants: c.209+1G>C (splicing defect) and c.980T>C (p. Leu327Leu). The *HADHA* gene did not contain potential pathogenic variants.

A pulmonologist was consulted because of the respiratory insufficiency during the first admission and complaints of shortness of breath during exercise. Pulmonary function showed slightly decreased vital capacity of 2.98 L (82% of predicted), normal maximum inspiratory pressure of 7.82 kPa (105% of predicted), and decreased maximum expiratory pressure of 4.62 kPa (49% of predicted), which was interpreted as decreased abdominal wall muscle strength accompanying MTP deficiency. Histamine provocation showed signs of bronchial hyper-reactivity, for which salbutamol and formoterol/beclomethasone were started.

Treatment for MTP deficiency was started with a long-chain fatty acids restricted, high carbohydrate and protein diet, supplemented with medium chain fatty acids, essential fatty acids, maltodextrin, and uncooked corn starch before bedtime. This improved her exercise endurance initially, but adherence to the diet proved difficult.

Discussion

Our case illustrates the difficult and long trajectory from first symptoms to the correct diagnosis of rare inborn errors of metabolism that can occur specifically in milder phenotypes of these diseases. MTP deficiency is a mitochondrial fatty acid β-oxidation disorder with a variable clinical phenotype. Timely diagnosis has important implications for management, mainly to prevent episodes of metabolic decompensation.

Although our patient had non-classified motor and sensory neuropathy discovered in childhood, and had been seen in our outpatient clinic months before, diagnosis of MTP deficiency was not made until she presented to our hospital with an episode of severe weakness and rhabdomyolysis, accompanying an Influenza B infection. Recording of the previous clinical history revealed that the patient

Table 1 Enzymatic activity measured in lymphocytes and fibroblasts

Cell type	LCHAD activity (nmol/(mg min protein))	Reference value	LCKAT activity (nmol/(mg min protein))	Reference value
Fibroblasts	12	34–114	6	58–110
Lymphocytes	6	22–74	2	23–43

LCHAD long-chain 3-hydroxyacyl-CoA dehydrogenase, *LCKAT* long-chain 3-ketoacyl-CoA thiolase

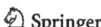

suffered from episodic weakness throughout her life triggered by gastroenteritis, fasting, and menstruation.

Nowadays, neonatal screening for MTP deficiency is performed by determination of the acylcarnitine profile in dried blood spots by tandem mass spectrometry. However, acylcarnitine profile can be completely normal when the test is performed in the absence of metabolic stress (Yagi et al. 2011), as was the case in our patient when her profile was tested 2 months after the second episode of rhabdomyolysis. As such, an earlier normal acylcarnitine profile, obtained as part of neonatal screening or otherwise, does not rule out the diagnosis of a long-chain fatty acid oxidation disorder in a patient that presents with symptoms fitting the diagnosis.

The clinical presentation, dominated by progressive peripheral neuropathy accompanied by episodic rhabdomyolysis, suggests that our patient suffered from the milder late-onset phenotype, which is most often caused by mutations in the *HADHA* gene. Sequence analysis, however, showed mutations in the *HADHB* gene, whereas previous case series showed that *HADHB* mutations are associated with phenotypes of either the severe neonatal form or the infantile hepatic form (Boutron et al. 2011). One of the variants (c.209+1G>C) demonstrated in our patient has previously been identified in a patient with a neonatal phenotype, who was homozygous for this mutation (Boutron et al. 2011). The second mutation (c.980T>C) has not been described earlier. It is possible that compound heterozygosity with the two described variants in our patient explains the MTP deficiency with a milder than expected phenotype. Compound heterozygosity has been described both in patients with *HADHA* gene mutations (Boutron et al. 2011), and in patients with *HADHB* gene mutations (Yagi et al. 2011).

A remarkable finding in our patient was a severe hypocalcaemia, caused by primary hypoparathyroidism. Although not a common feature of MTP deficiency, (congenital) hypoparathyroidism has been reported in five patients before (Dionisi-Vici et al. 2003; Tyni et al. 1997; Labarthe et al. 2006; Naiki et al. 2014). In four patients, including two siblings, MTP deficiency was caused by mutations in the *HADHB* gene (Dionisi-Vici et al. 2003; Labarthe et al. 2006; Naiki et al. 2014), whereas one patient had isolated LCHAD deficiency (Tyni et al. 1997). All four patients with MTP deficiency showed a clinical picture similar to our patient, dominated by distal peripheral neuropathy with lower limb weakness, and episodic rhabdomyolysis triggered by (viral) infections and fasting. Although hypocalcaemia is frequently observed during rhabdomyolysis due to renal failure, in our patient kidney function remained normal and PTH was low during both admissions. Moreover, the patient's medical history reported hypoparathyroidism earlier on in life. The pathophysiological link between (congenital) hypoparathyroidism and MTP deficiency is unclear. It has been suggested that mutations in enzymes involved in the β-oxidation of fatty acids cause congenital malformation leading to absence of parathyroid glands (Tyni et al. 1997). However, since all other organs develop normally this is not a very likely explanation. In some reported patients and in our patient, there was partial recovery of parathyroid function following treatment, suggesting parathyroid hypoplasia or impaired secretion of PTH (Labarthe et al. 2006). Others suggested that the accumulation of long-chain fatty acids in parathyroid glands could cause direct cellular toxicity (Saudubray et al. 1999). This may explain why PTH is lower at the time of metabolic decompensation.

Our case underlines the importance of determination of an acylcarnitine profile in adult patients with unexplained peripheral neuropathy, when this is accompanied by episodic exacerbations of weakness, exercise intolerance, or documented rhabdomyolysis. Recording of the previous clinical history should focus on known triggers, such as fasting or infections. Metabolic screening should preferably be performed during these exacerbations, since screening may be unremarkable in patients with MTP deficiency in absence of high metabolic demand. Lastly, primary (congenital) hypoparathyroidism may be a feature of MTP deficiency and could be the initial presentation of the disease in infancy.

Synopsis

Mitochondrial trifunctional protein deficiency can present as a cluster of peripheral neuropathy, hypoparathyroidism, and episodic exacerbations during metabolic stress, with the important notice that metabolic screening may be normal when performed when no metabolic stress is present.

Compliance with Ethics Guidelines

Author Contributions

All authors were involved in drafting the manuscript and revising it critically for important intellectual content and have agreed upon submission of the manuscript.

Competing Interest/Funding

Peter van Vliet, Annelies Berden, Mojca van Schie, Jaap Bakker, Christian Heringhaus, Irenaeus de Coo, Mirjam

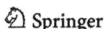

Langeveld, Marielle Schroijen, and Sesmu Arbous declare that they have no conflicts of interest. This case report was not supported by any funding source.

Ethics Approval/Consent

This case report did not need evaluation by a medical ethical committee. Informed consent to publish the case report was obtained from the patient.

References

Boutron A, Acquaviva C, Vianey-Saban C et al (2011) Comprehensive cDNA study and quantitative analysis of mutant HADHA and HADHB transcripts in a French cohort of 52 patients with mitochondrial trifunctional protein deficiency. Mol Genet Metabol 103:341–348

Brackett JC, Sims HF, Rinaldo P et al (1995) Two α-subunit donor splice site mutations cause human trifunctional protein deficiency. J Clin Invest 95:2076–2082

Dionisi-Vici C, Garavaglia B, Burlina AB et al (2003) Hypoparathyroidism in mitochondrial trifunctional protein deficiency. J Pediatr 129:159–162

Labarthe F, Benoist JF, Brivet M, Vianey-Saban C, Despert F, Ogier de Baulny H (2006) Partial hypoparathyroidism associated with mitochondrial trifunctional protein deficiency. Eur J Pediatr 165:389–391

Morris AM, Spiekerkoetter U (2016) Disorders of mitochondrial fatty acid oxidation & riboflavin metabolism. In: Saudubray J-M et al (eds) Inborn metabolic diseases. Springer-Verlag, Berlin Heidelberg, pp 201–213

Naiki M, Ochi N, Kato YS et al (2014) Mutations in HADHB, which encodes the β-subunit of mitochondrial trifunctional protein, cause infantile onset hypoparathyroidism and peripheral polyneuropathy. Am J Med Genet A 164A:1180–1187

Sander J, Sander S, Steuerwald U et al (2005) Neonatal screening for defects of the mitochondrial trifunctional protein. Mol Genet Metabol 85:108–114

Saudubray JM, Martin D, de Lonlay P et al (1999) Recognition and management of fatty acid oxidation defects: a series of 107 patients. J Inherit Metab Dis 22:488–502

Spiekerkoetter U, Sun B, Khuchua Z, Bennet MJ, Strauss AJ (2003a) Molecular and phenotypic heterogeneity in mitochondrial trifunctional protein deficiency due to β-subunit mutations. Hum Mutat 21:598–607

Spiekerkoetter U, Khuchua Z, Yue Z, Bennett MJ, Strauss AW (2003b) General mitochondrial trifunctional protein (TFP) deficiency as a result of either α- or β-subunit mutations exhibits similar phenotypes because mutations in either subunit alter TFP complex expression and subunit turnover. Pediatr Res 55:190–196

Tyni T, Rapola J, Palotie A, Pikho H (1997) Hypoparathyroidism in a patient with long-chain-3-hydroxyacyl-coenzyme-A de hydrogenase deficiency caused by the G1528C mutation. J Pediatr 131:766–768

Yagi M, Lee T, Awano H et al (2011) A patient with mitochondrial trifunctional protein deficiency due to the mutations in the HADHB gene showed recurrent myalgia since early childhood and was diagnosed in adolescence. Mol Genet Metabol 104:556–559

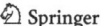